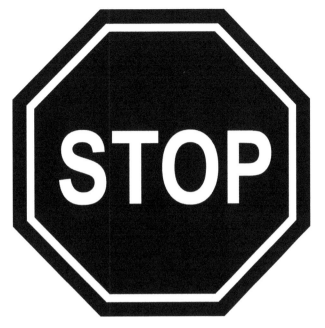

FREE Test Taking Tips Video/DVD Offer

To better serve you, we created videos covering test taking tips that we want to give you for FREE. **These videos cover world-class tips that will help you succeed on your test.**

We just ask that you send us feedback about this product. Please let us know what you thought about it—whether good, bad, or indifferent.

To get your **FREE videos**, you can use the QR code below or email freevideos@studyguideteam.com with "Free Videos" in the subject line and the following information in the body of the email:

>   a. The title of your product

>   b. Your product rating on a scale of 1-5, with 5 being the highest

>   c. Your feedback about the product

If you have any questions or concerns, please don't hesitate to contact us at info@studyguideteam.com.

Thank you!

MBLEx Study Guide 2022 - 2023

MBLEx Test Prep with Practice Exam Questions for the FSMTB Certification [9th Edition]

Joshua Rueda

Interested in buying more than 10 copies of our product? Contact us about bulk discounts:
bulkorders@studyguideteam.com

ISBN 13: 9781637754948
ISBN 10: 1637754949

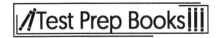

Table of Contents

Quick Overview

As you draw closer to taking your exam, effective preparation becomes more and more important. Thankfully, you have this study guide to help you get ready. Use this guide to help keep your studying on track and refer to it often.

This study guide contains several key sections that will help you be successful on your exam. The guide contains tips for what you should do the night before and the day of the test. Also included are test-taking tips. Knowing the right information is not always enough. Many well-prepared test takers struggle with exams. These tips will help equip you to accurately read, assess, and answer test questions.

A large part of the guide is devoted to showing you what content to expect on the exam and to helping you better understand that content. In this guide are practice test questions so that you can see how well you have grasped the content. Then, answer explanations are provided so that you can understand why you missed certain questions.

Don't try to cram the night before you take your exam. This is not a wise strategy for a few reasons. First, your retention of the information will be low. Your time would be better used by reviewing information you already know rather than trying to learn a lot of new information. Second, you will likely become stressed as you try to gain a large amount of knowledge in a short amount of time. Third, you will be depriving yourself of sleep. So be sure to go to bed at a reasonable time the night before. Being well-rested helps you focus and remain calm.

Be sure to eat a substantial breakfast the morning of the exam. If you are taking the exam in the afternoon, be sure to have a good lunch as well. Being hungry is distracting and can make it difficult to focus. You have hopefully spent lots of time preparing for the exam. Don't let an empty stomach get in the way of success!

When travelling to the testing center, leave earlier than needed. That way, you have a buffer in case you experience any delays. This will help you remain calm and will keep you from missing your appointment time at the testing center.

Be sure to pace yourself during the exam. Don't try to rush through the exam. There is no need to risk performing poorly on the exam just so you can leave the testing center early. Allow yourself to use all of the allotted time if needed.

Remain positive while taking the exam even if you feel like you are performing poorly. Thinking about the content you should have mastered will not help you perform better on the exam.

Once the exam is complete, take some time to relax. Even if you feel that you need to take the exam again, you will be well served by some down time before you begin studying again. It's often easier to convince yourself to study if you know that it will come with a reward!

Test-Taking Strategies

1. Predicting the Answer

When you feel confident in your preparation for a multiple-choice test, try predicting the answer before reading the answer choices. This is especially useful on questions that test objective factual knowledge. By predicting the answer before reading the available choices, you eliminate the possibility that you will be distracted or led astray by an incorrect answer choice. You will feel more confident in your selection if you read the question, predict the answer, and then find your prediction among the answer choices. After using this strategy, be sure to still read all of the answer choices carefully and completely. If you feel unprepared, you should not attempt to predict the answers. This would be a waste of time and an opportunity for your mind to wander in the wrong direction.

2. Reading the Whole Question

Too often, test takers scan a multiple-choice question, recognize a few familiar words, and immediately jump to the answer choices. Test authors are aware of this common impatience, and they will sometimes prey upon it. For instance, a test author might subtly turn the question into a negative, or he or she might redirect the focus of the question right at the end. The only way to avoid falling into these traps is to read the entirety of the question carefully before reading the answer choices.

3. Looking for Wrong Answers

Long and complicated multiple-choice questions can be intimidating. One way to simplify a difficult multiple-choice question is to eliminate all of the answer choices that are clearly wrong. In most sets of answers, there will be at least one selection that can be dismissed right away. If the test is administered on paper, the test taker could draw a line through it to indicate that it may be ignored; otherwise, the test taker will have to perform this operation mentally or on scratch paper. In either case, once the obviously incorrect answers have been eliminated, the remaining choices may be considered. Sometimes identifying the clearly wrong answers will give the test taker some information about the correct answer. For instance, if one of the remaining answer choices is a direct opposite of one of the eliminated answer choices, it may well be the correct answer. The opposite of obviously wrong is obviously right! Of course, this is not always the case. Some answers are obviously incorrect simply because they are irrelevant to the question being asked. Still, identifying and eliminating some incorrect answer choices is a good way to simplify a multiple-choice question.

4. Don't Overanalyze

Anxious test takers often overanalyze questions. When you are nervous, your brain will often run wild, causing you to make associations and discover clues that don't actually exist. If you feel that this may be a problem for you, do whatever you can to slow down during the test. Try taking a deep breath or counting to ten. As you read and consider the question, restrict yourself to the particular words used by the author. Avoid thought tangents about what the author *really* meant, or what he or she was *trying* to say. The only things that matter on a multiple-choice test are the words that are actually in the question. You must avoid reading too much into a multiple-choice question, or supposing that the writer meant something other than what he or she wrote.

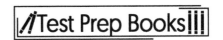

5. No Need for Panic

It is wise to learn as many strategies as possible before taking a multiple-choice test, but it is likely that you will come across a few questions for which you simply don't know the answer. In this situation, avoid panicking. Because most multiple-choice tests include dozens of questions, the relative value of a single wrong answer is small. As much as possible, you should compartmentalize each question on a multiple-choice test. In other words, you should not allow your feelings about one question to affect your success on the others. When you find a question that you either don't understand or don't know how to answer, just take a deep breath and do your best. Read the entire question slowly and carefully. Try rephrasing the question a couple of different ways. Then, read all of the answer choices carefully. After eliminating obviously wrong answers, make a selection and move on to the next question.

6. Confusing Answer Choices

When working on a difficult multiple-choice question, there may be a tendency to focus on the answer choices that are the easiest to understand. Many people, whether consciously or not, gravitate to the answer choices that require the least concentration, knowledge, and memory. This is a mistake. When you come across an answer choice that is confusing, you should give it extra attention. A question might be confusing because you do not know the subject matter to which it refers. If this is the case, don't eliminate the answer before you have affirmatively settled on another. When you come across an answer choice of this type, set it aside as you look at the remaining choices. If you can confidently assert that one of the other choices is correct, you can leave the confusing answer aside. Otherwise, you will need to take a moment to try to better understand the confusing answer choice. Rephrasing is one way to tease out the sense of a confusing answer choice.

7. Your First Instinct

Many people struggle with multiple-choice tests because they overthink the questions. If you have studied sufficiently for the test, you should be prepared to trust your first instinct once you have carefully and completely read the question and all of the answer choices. There is a great deal of research suggesting that the mind can come to the correct conclusion very quickly once it has obtained all of the relevant information. At times, it may seem to you as if your intuition is working faster even than your reasoning mind. This may in fact be true. The knowledge you obtain while studying may be retrieved from your subconscious before you have a chance to work out the associations that support it. Verify your instinct by working out the reasons that it should be trusted.

8. Key Words

Many test takers struggle with multiple-choice questions because they have poor reading comprehension skills. Quickly reading and understanding a multiple-choice question requires a mixture of skill and experience. To help with this, try jotting down a few key words and phrases on a piece of scrap paper. Doing this concentrates the process of reading and forces the mind to weigh the relative importance of the question's parts. In selecting words and phrases to write down, the test taker thinks about the question more deeply and carefully. This is especially true for multiple-choice questions that are preceded by a long prompt.

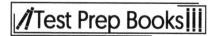

9. Subtle Negatives

One of the oldest tricks in the multiple-choice test writer's book is to subtly reverse the meaning of a question with a word like *not* or *except*. If you are not paying attention to each word in the question, you can easily be led astray by this trick. For instance, a common question format is, "Which of the following is...?" Obviously, if the question instead is, "Which of the following is not...?," then the answer will be quite different. Even worse, the test makers are aware of the potential for this mistake and will include one answer choice that would be correct if the question were not negated or reversed. A test taker who misses the reversal will find what he or she believes to be a correct answer and will be so confident that he or she will fail to reread the question and discover the original error. The only way to avoid this is to practice a wide variety of multiple-choice questions and to pay close attention to each and every word.

10. Reading Every Answer Choice

It may seem obvious, but you should always read every one of the answer choices! Too many test takers fall into the habit of scanning the question and assuming that they understand the question because they recognize a few key words. From there, they pick the first answer choice that answers the question they believe they have read. Test takers who read all of the answer choices might discover that one of the latter answer choices is actually *more* correct. Moreover, reading all of the answer choices can remind you of facts related to the question that can help you arrive at the correct answer. Sometimes, a misstatement or incorrect detail in one of the latter answer choices will trigger your memory of the subject and will enable you to find the right answer. Failing to read all of the answer choices is like not reading all of the items on a restaurant menu: you might miss out on the perfect choice.

11. Spot the Hedges

One of the keys to success on multiple-choice tests is paying close attention to every word. This is never truer than with words like almost, most, some, and sometimes. These words are called "hedges" because they indicate that a statement is not totally true or not true in every place and time. An absolute statement will contain no hedges, but in many subjects, the answers are not always straightforward or absolute. There are always exceptions to the rules in these subjects. For this reason, you should favor those multiple-choice questions that contain hedging language. The presence of qualifying words indicates that the author is taking special care with their words, which is certainly important when composing the right answer. After all, there are many ways to be wrong, but there is only one way to be right! For this reason, it is wise to avoid answers that are absolute when taking a multiple-choice test. An absolute answer is one that says things are either all one way or all another. They often include words like *every*, *always*, *best*, and *never*. If you are taking a multiple-choice test in a subject that doesn't lend itself to absolute answers, be on your guard if you see any of these words.

12. Long Answers

In many subject areas, the answers are not simple. As already mentioned, the right answer often requires hedges. Another common feature of the answers to a complex or subjective question are qualifying clauses, which are groups of words that subtly modify the meaning of the sentence. If the question or answer choice describes a rule to which there are exceptions or the subject matter is complicated, ambiguous, or confusing, the correct answer will require many words in order to be expressed clearly and accurately. In essence, you should not be deterred by answer choices that seem

4

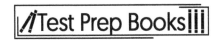

excessively long. Oftentimes, the author of the text will not be able to write the correct answer without offering some qualifications and modifications. Your job is to read the answer choices thoroughly and completely and to select the one that most accurately and precisely answers the question.

13. Restating to Understand

Sometimes, a question on a multiple-choice test is difficult not because of what it asks but because of how it is written. If this is the case, restate the question or answer choice in different words. This process serves a couple of important purposes. First, it forces you to concentrate on the core of the question. In order to rephrase the question accurately, you have to understand it well. Rephrasing the question will concentrate your mind on the key words and ideas. Second, it will present the information to your mind in a fresh way. This process may trigger your memory and render some useful scrap of information picked up while studying.

14. True Statements

Sometimes an answer choice will be true in itself, but it does not answer the question. This is one of the main reasons why it is essential to read the question carefully and completely before proceeding to the answer choices. Too often, test takers skip ahead to the answer choices and look for true statements. Having found one of these, they are content to select it without reference to the question above. Obviously, this provides an easy way for test makers to play tricks. The savvy test taker will always read the entire question before turning to the answer choices. Then, having settled on a correct answer choice, he or she will refer to the original question and ensure that the selected answer is relevant. The mistake of choosing a correct-but-irrelevant answer choice is especially common on questions related to specific pieces of objective knowledge. A prepared test taker will have a wealth of factual knowledge at their disposal and should not be careless in its application.

15. No Patterns

One of the more dangerous ideas that circulates about multiple-choice tests is that the correct answers tend to fall into patterns. These erroneous ideas range from a belief that B and C are the most common right answers, to the idea that an unprepared test-taker should answer "A-B-A-C-A-D-A-B-A." It cannot be emphasized enough that pattern-seeking of this type is exactly the WRONG way to approach a multiple-choice test. To begin with, it is highly unlikely that the test maker will plot the correct answers according to some predetermined pattern. The questions are scrambled and delivered in a random order. Furthermore, even if the test maker was following a pattern in the assignation of correct answers, there is no reason why the test taker would know which pattern he or she was using. Any attempt to discern a pattern in the answer choices is a waste of time and a distraction from the real work of taking the test. A test taker would be much better served by extra preparation before the test than by reliance on a pattern in the answers.

FREE Videos/DVD OFFER

Doing well on your exam requires both knowing the test content and understanding how to use that knowledge to do well on the test. We offer completely FREE test taking tip videos. **These videos cover world-class tips that you can use to succeed on your test.**

To get your **FREE videos**, you can use the QR code below or email freevideos@studyguideteam.com with "Free Videos" in the subject line and the following information in the body of the email:

    a. The title of your product

    b. Your product rating on a scale of 1-5, with 5 being the highest

    c. Your feedback about the product

If you have any questions or concerns, please don't hesitate to contact us at info@studyguideteam.com.

Thanks again!

Introduction to the MBLEx

Function of the Test

The Massage & Bodywork Licensing Examination (MBLEx, pronounced "EM-blex") is part of the entry-level licensing process for aspiring massage therapists in forty-two states (Vermont, Minnesota, Wyoming, Kansas, and Oklahoma are not regulated; Hawaii, New York, and Massachusetts are regulated but do not use the test), the District of Columbia, Puerto Rico, and the U.S. Virgin Islands. A competing exam, the NCBTMB, was accepted by most of these states until 2014, when the NCBTMB was discontinued.

The MBLEx was created by the Federation of State Massage Therapy Boards (FSMTB) in 2007 and has been operated by the FSMTB since that year. While some employers request and consider scores on the MBLEx, it is primarily used only in the licensing process. Accordingly, most test takers are young, prospective professional massage therapists engaged in or having recently completed an educational massage therapy program.

Test Administration

The MBLEx is offered daily, year-round, exclusively by computer at Pearson VUE test centers throughout the U.S. and its territories. The test fee is $195 for the first attempt and the same amount for any subsequent retakes. This amount will change to $265 starting April 1, 2020. The FSMTB permits students to retake the exam any time after thirty days have elapsed since a previous attempt, but individual state licensing boards may have rules that further restrict retesting.

The test is administered in both English and Spanish. Pursuant to the ADA, the FSMTB will review requests from qualified candidates with diagnosed disabilities and accommodate those it deems reasonable and not unnecessarily disruptive.

People wishing to take the test must apply for and receive an Authorization to Test (ATT), at which point they will have a ninety-day window in which to schedule and take the exam.

Test Format

The test lasts 110 minutes and is comprised of one hundred multiple-choice questions, each with four answer options. Questions may not be skipped, and must instead be answered in the order presented.

The material on the MBLEx is based on a Job Task Analysis covering the experiences of professional massage therapists. The content currently on the exam is based on a 2017 analysis.

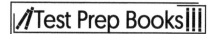

The content comprises eight categories as detailed below:

Category	Share of Test
Anatomy & Physiology	11%
Kinesiology	12%
Pathology, Contraindications, Areas of Caution, Special Populations	14%
Benefits and Physiological Effects of Techniques that Manipulate Soft Tissue	15%
Client Assessment, Reassessment, & Treatment Planning	17%
Ethics, Boundaries, Laws, Regulations	16%
Guidelines for Professional Practice	15%

Scoring

The test is adaptive, which means that the difficulty of questions given to the test taker get harder if they perform well and get easier if they perform poorly. The test taker's score is based on both the number of questions they get right and also the difficulty of those questions. There is no penalty for guessing.

The total scaled score on the MBLEx ranges from 300 to 900. A scaled score of 630 is required to pass. Students that pass will receive a score report indicating that they have passed, while students that fail will receive diagnostic information indicating which areas they performed well and poorly on.

Recent/Future Developments

The new version of the MBLEx, implemented beginning July 2018, eliminates the previous section entitled "Overview of Massage/Bodywork Modalities, History and Culture." Instead, the Overview of Massage/Bodywork Modalities content is migrated to the "Benefits and Physiological Effects of Techniques that Manipulate Soft Tissue" section. The exam no longer assesses the test taker's knowledge of the "History and Culture" of massage. These changes slightly alter the percentage contribution that the remaining seven categories now carry, as the 5% of the questions that the eliminated eighth section had contributed is now redistributed. For example, the "Guidelines for Professional Practice" section changes from 13% to 15% of the total test questions.

Study Prep Plan for the MBLEX

1   **Schedule -** Use one of our study schedules below or come up with one of your own.

2   **Relax -** Test anxiety can hurt even the best students. There are many ways to reduce stress. Find the one that works best for you.

3   **Execute -** Once you have a good plan in place, be sure to stick to it.

One Week Study Schedule		
Day 1	Anatomy and Physiology	
Day 2	Pathology, Contraindications, Areas of...	
Day 3	Benefits and Physiological Effects of...	
Day 4	Ethics, Boundaries, Laws & Regulations	
Day 5	Practice Tests #1 & #2	
Day 6	Practice Test #3	
Day 7	Take Your Exam!	

Two Week Study Schedule			
Day 1	Anatomy and Physiology	Day 8	Practice Test #1
Day 2	Kinesiology	Day 9	Answer Explanations #1
Day 3	Pathology, Contraindications...	Day 10	Practice Test #2
Day 4	Benefits and Physiological Effects of...	Day 11	Answer Explanations #2
Day 5	Client Assessment, Reassessment, and...	Day 12	Practice Test #3
Day 6	Ethics, Boundaries, Laws & Regulations	Day 13	Answer Explanations #3
Day 7	Guidelines for Professional Practice	Day 14	Take Your Exam!

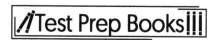

One Month Study Schedule					
Day 1	Anatomy and Physiology	Day 11	Classes of Medications	Day 21	Guidelines for Professional Practice
Day 2	Endocrine System Structure and Function	Day 12	Practice Questions	Day 22	Business Practices
Day 3	Reproductive System Structure and Function	Day 13	Benefits and Physiological Effects of Techniques that...	Day 23	Practice Questions
Day 4	Levels of Organization of the Human Body	Day 14	Overview of Massage/ Bodywork Modalities	Day 24	Practice Test #1
Day 5	Practice Questions	Day 15	Practice Questions	Day 25	Answer Explanations #1
Day 6	Kinesiology	Day 16	Client Assessment, Reassessment, and...	Day 26	Practice Test #2
Day 7	Locations, Attachments, and Actions of Muscles	Day 17	Practice Questions	Day 27	Answer Explanations #2
Day 8	Practice Questions	Day 18	Ethics, Boundaries, Laws & Regulations	Day 28	Practice Test #3
Day 9	Pathology, Contraindications, Areas of Caution...	Day 19	Scope of Practice	Day 29	Answer Explanations #3
Day 10	Contraindications	Day 20	Practice Questions	Day 30	Take Your Exam!

Build your own prep plan by visiting:
testprepbooks.com/prep

Anatomy and Physiology

Anatomy is the structural makeup of an organism. The study of anatomy may be divided into microscopic/fine anatomy and macroscopic/gross anatomy. Fine anatomy concerns itself with viewing the features of the body with the aid of a microscope, while gross anatomy concerns itself with viewing the features of the body with the naked eye. **Physiology** refers to the functions of an organism, and it examines the chemical or physical functions that help the body function appropriately. Successful massage therapists must have a foundational understanding of anatomy and physiology in order to deliver safe, effective treatments to clients.

Circulatory System Structure and Function

The **circulatory system** is a network of organs and tubes that transport blood, hormones, nutrients, oxygen, and other gases to cells and tissues throughout the body. It is also known as the **cardiovascular system**. The major components of the circulatory system are the blood vessels, blood, and heart.

Blood Vessels

In the circulatory system, **blood vessels** are responsible for transporting blood throughout the body. The three major types of blood vessels in the circulatory system are arteries, veins, and capillaries. **Arteries** carry blood from the heart to the rest of the body. Veins carry blood from the body back to the heart. **Capillaries** connect arteries to veins and form networks that exchange materials between the blood and the cells.

In general, arteries are stronger and thicker than veins, as they withstand high pressures exerted by the blood as the heart pumps it through the body. Arteries control blood flow through either **vasoconstriction** (narrowing of the blood vessel's diameter) or **vasodilation** (widening of the blood vessel's diameter). The blood in veins is under much lower pressures, so veins have valves to prevent the backflow of blood.

Most of the exchange between the blood and tissues takes place through the capillaries. There are three types of capillaries: continuous, fenestrated, and sinusoidal.

Continuous capillaries are made up of epithelial cells tightly connected together. As a result, they limit the types of materials that pass into and out of the blood. Continuous capillaries are the most common type of capillary. **Fenestrated capillaries** have openings that allow materials to be freely exchanged between the blood and tissues. They are commonly found in the digestive, endocrine, and urinary systems. **Sinusoidal capillaries** have larger openings and allow proteins and blood cells through. They are found primarily in the liver, bone marrow, and spleen.

Blood

Blood is vital to the human body. It is a liquid connective tissue that serves as a transport system for supplying cells with nutrients and carrying away their wastes. The average adult human has five to six quarts of blood circulating through their body. Approximately 55% of blood is **plasma** (the fluid portion), and the remaining 45% is composed of solid cells and cell parts.

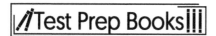
There are three major types of blood cells:

- **Red blood cells**, or **erythrocytes**, transport oxygen throughout the body. They contain a protein called **hemoglobin** that allows them to carry oxygen. The iron in the hemoglobin gives the cells and the blood their red colors.

- **White blood cells**, or **leukocytes,** are responsible for fighting infectious diseases and maintaining the immune system. There are five types of white blood cells: neutrophils, lymphocytes, eosinophils, monocytes, and basophils.

- **Platelets** are cell fragments that play a central role in the blood clotting process.

All blood cells in adults are produced in the bone marrow—red blood cells and most white blood cells are produced in the red marrow, and some white blood cells are produced in the yellow bone marrow.

Heart

The heart is a two-part, muscular pump that forcefully pushes blood throughout the human body. The human heart has four chambers—two upper **atria** and two lower **ventricles** separated by a partition called the septum. There is a pair on the left and a pair on the right. Anatomically, *left* and *right* correspond to the sides of the body that the individual themselves would refer to as left and right.

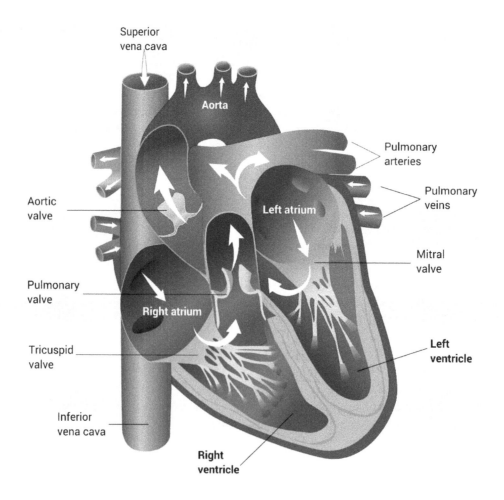

12

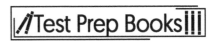

Four valves help to section off the chambers from one another. Between the right atrium and ventricle, the three flaps of the **tricuspid valve** keep blood from flowing backwards from the ventricle to the atrium, similar to how the two flaps of the **mitral valve** work between the left atrium and ventricle. As these two valves lie between an atrium and a ventricle, they are referred to as atrioventricular (AV) valves. The other two valves are **semilunar (SL)** and they control blood flow into the two great arteries leaving the ventricles. The **pulmonary valve** connects the right ventricle to the pulmonary artery, while the **aortic valve** connects the left ventricle to the aorta.

Cardiac Cycle

A **cardiac cycle** is one complete sequence of cardiac activity. The cardiac cycle represents the relaxation and contraction of the heart and can be divided into two phases: diastole and systole.

Diastole is the phase during which the heart relaxes and fills with blood. It gives rise to the **diastolic blood pressure (DBP)**, which is the bottom number of a blood pressure reading. **Systole** is the phase during which the heart contracts and discharges blood. It gives rise to the **systolic blood pressure (SBP)**, which is the top number of a blood pressure reading. The heart's electrical conduction system coordinates the cardiac cycle.

Types of Circulation

Five major blood vessels manage blood flow to and from the heart: the superior and inferior venae cava, the aorta, the pulmonary artery, and the pulmonary vein.

The **superior vena cava** is a large vein that drains blood from the head and the upper body. The **inferior vena cava** is a large vein that drains blood from the lower body. The **aorta** is the largest artery in the human body and carries blood from the heart to body tissues. The **pulmonary arteries** carry blood from the heart to the lungs. The **pulmonary veins** transport blood from the lungs to the heart.

In the human body, there are two types of circulation: pulmonary circulation and systemic circulation. **Pulmonary circulation** supplies blood to the lungs. Deoxygenated blood enters the right atrium of the heart and is routed through the tricuspid valve into the right ventricle. Deoxygenated blood then travels from the right ventricle of the heart through the pulmonary valve and into the pulmonary arteries. The pulmonary arteries carry the deoxygenated blood to the lungs. In the lungs, oxygen is absorbed, and carbon dioxide is released. The pulmonary veins carry oxygenated blood to the left atrium of the heart.

Systemic circulation supplies blood to all other parts of the body, except the lungs. Oxygenated blood flows from the left atrium of the heart through the mitral, or bicuspid, valve into the left ventricle of the heart. Oxygenated blood is then routed from the left ventricle of the heart through the aortic valve and into the aorta. The aorta delivers blood to the systemic arteries, which supply the body tissues. In the tissues, oxygen and nutrients are exchanged for carbon dioxide and other wastes. The deoxygenated blood along with carbon dioxide and wastes enter the systemic veins, where they are returned to the right atrium of the heart via the superior and inferior vena cava.

Digestive System Structure and Function

The human body relies completely on the digestive system to meet its nutritional needs. After food and drink are ingested, the **digestive system** breaks them down into their component nutrients and absorbs them so that the circulatory system can transport the nutrients to other cells to use for growth, energy,

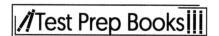
and cell repair. These nutrients may be classified as proteins, lipids, carbohydrates, vitamins, and minerals.

The digestive system is thought of chiefly in two parts: the **digestive tract** (also called the **alimentary tract** or **gastrointestinal tract**) and the accessory digestive organs. The digestive tract is the pathway in which food is ingested, digested, absorbed, and excreted. It is composed of the mouth, pharynx, esophagus, stomach, small and large intestines, rectum, and anus. **Peristalsis,** or wave-like contractions of smooth muscle, moves food and wastes through the digestive tract. The **accessory digestive organs** are the salivary glands, liver, gallbladder, and pancreas.

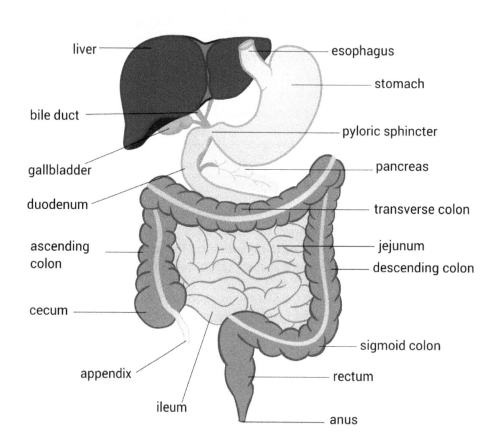

Mouth and Stomach

The **mouth** is the entrance to the digestive system. Here, the mechanical and chemical digestion of the food begins. The food is chewed mechanically by the teeth and shaped into a **bolus** by the tongue so that it can be more easily swallowed by the esophagus. The food also becomes waterier and more pliable with the addition of saliva secreted from the **salivary glands**, the largest of which are the **parotid glands**. The glands also secrete **amylase** in the saliva, an enzyme that begins chemical digestion and breakdown of the carbohydrates and sugars in the food.

The food then moves through the **pharynx** and down the muscular **esophagus** to the stomach.

14

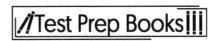

The **stomach** is a large, muscular sac-like organ at the distal end of the esophagus. Here, the bolus is subjected to more mechanical and chemical digestion. As it passes through the stomach, it is physically squeezed and crushed while additional secretions turn it into a watery nutrient-filled liquid that exits into the small intestine as **chyme**.

The stomach secretes many substances into the **lumen** of the digestive tract. Some cells produce **gastrin**, a hormone that prompts other cells in the stomach to secrete a gastric acid composed mostly of hydrochloric acid (HCl). The HCl is at such a high concentration and low pH that it denatures most proteins and degrades a lot of organic matter. The stomach also secretes mucous to form a protective film that keeps the corrosive acid from dissolving its own cells; gaps in this mucous layer can lead to peptic ulcers. Finally, the stomach also uses digestive enzymes like **proteases** and **lipases** to break down proteins and fats; although there are some gastric lipases here, the stomach mostly breaks down proteins.

Small Intestine

The chyme from the stomach enters the first part of the small intestine, the **duodenum,** through the **pyloric sphincter**, and its extreme acidity is partly neutralized by sodium bicarbonate secreted along with mucous. The presence of chyme in the duodenum triggers the secretion of the hormones secretin and cholecystokinin (CCK). **Secretin** acts on the pancreas to dump more sodium bicarbonate into the small intestine so that the pH is kept at a reasonable level, while **CCK** acts on the gallbladder to release the *bile* that it has been storing. **Bile,** a substance produced by the liver and stored in the gallbladder, helps to **emulsify** or dissolve fats and lipids.

Because of the bile, which aids in lipid absorption, and the secreted **lipases**, which break down fats, the duodenum is the chief site of fat digestion in the body. The duodenum also represents the last major site of chemical digestion in the digestive tract, as the other two sections of the small intestine (the **jejunum** and **ileum**) are instead heavily involved in absorption of nutrients.

The small intestine reaches 40 feet in length, and its cells are arranged in small finger-like projections called **villi**. This is due to its key role in the absorption of nearly all nutrients from the ingested and digested food, effectively transferring them from the lumen of the GI tract to the bloodstream, where they travel to the cells that need them. These nutrients include simple sugars like glucose from carbohydrates, amino acids from proteins, emulsified fats, electrolytes like sodium and potassium, minerals like iron and zinc, and vitamins like D and B12. Vitamin B12's absorption, though it takes place in the intestines, is actually aided by **intrinsic factor** that was released into the chyme back in the stomach.

Large Intestine

The leftover parts of food which remain unabsorbed or undigested in the lumen of the small intestine next travel through the **large intestine**, that may also be referred to as the **large bowel** or **colon**. The large intestine is mainly responsible for water absorption. As the chyme at this stage no longer has any useful nutrients that can be absorbed by the body, it is now referred to as **waste**, and it is stored in the large intestine until it can be excreted from the body. Removing the liquid from the waste transforms it from liquid to solid stool, or **feces**.

This waste first passes from the small intestine to the **cecum**, a pouch that forms the first part of the large intestine. In herbivores, it provides a place for bacteria to digest cellulose, but in humans most of it is vestigial and is known as the **appendix**. The appendix has no known function other than arbitrarily

15

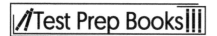

becoming inflamed. From the cecum, waste next travels up the ascending colon, across the transverse colon, down the descending colon, and through the sigmoid colon to the rectum. The **rectum** is responsible for the final storage of waste before it is expelled through the **anus**. The **anal canal** is a small portion of the rectum leading through to the anus and the outside of the body.

Pancreas

The **pancreas** has endocrine and exocrine functions. The endocrine function works to regulate blood sugar levels. It involves releasing the hormone **insulin,** which decreases blood sugar (glucose) levels, or **glucagon**, which increases blood sugar (glucose) levels, directly into the bloodstream. Both hormones are produced in the **islets of Langerhans**, insulin in the **beta cells** and glucagon in the **alpha cells**.

The major part of the gland has an exocrine function, which consists of acinar cells secreting inactive digestive enzymes (**zymogens**) into the main pancreatic duct. The main pancreatic duct joins the common bile duct, which empties into the small intestine (specifically the duodenum). The digestive enzymes are then activated and take part in the digestion of carbohydrates, proteins, and fats within **chyme** (the mixture of partially digested food and digestive juices).

Endocrine System Structure and Function

The **endocrine system** is made of the ductless tissues and glands that secrete hormones into the interstitial fluids of the body. **Interstitial fluid** is the solution that surrounds tissue cells within the body. This system works closely with the nervous system to regulate the physiological activities of the other systems of the body to maintain homeostasis. While the nervous system provides quick, short-term responses to stimuli, the endocrine system acts by releasing hormones into the bloodstream that get distributed to the whole body. The response is slow but long-lasting, ranging from a few hours to a few weeks.

Hormones are chemical substances that change the metabolic activity of tissues and organs. While regular metabolic reactions are controlled by enzymes, hormones can change the type, activity, or quantity of the enzymes involved in the reaction. They bind to specific cells and start a biochemical chain of events that changes the enzymatic activity. Hormones can regulate development and growth, digestive metabolism, mood, and body temperature, among other things. Often small amounts of hormone will lead to large changes in the body.

The endocrine system has the following major glands:

- **Hypothalamus:** A part of the brain, the hypothalamus connects the nervous system to the endocrine system via the pituitary gland. Although it is considered part of the nervous system, it plays a dual role in regulating endocrine organs.

- **Pituitary Gland:** A pea-sized gland found at the bottom of the hypothalamus. It has two lobes, called the anterior and posterior lobes. It plays an important role in regulating the function of other endocrine glands. The hormones released control growth, blood pressure, certain functions of the sex organs, salt concentration of the kidneys, internal temperature regulation, and pain relief.

- **Thyroid Gland:** This gland releases hormones, such as thyroxine, that are important for metabolism, growth and development, temperature regulation, and brain development during

16

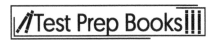

infancy and childhood. Thyroid hormones also monitor the amount of circulating calcium in the body.

- **Parathyroid Glands:** These are four pea-sized glands located on the posterior surface of the thyroid. The main hormone secreted is called **parathyroid hormone (PTH)** and helps with the thyroid's regulation of calcium in the body.

- **Thymus Gland:** The thymus is located in the chest cavity, embedded in connective tissue. It produces several hormones important for development and maintenance of normal immunological defenses. One hormone promotes the development and maturation of lymphocytes, which strengthens the immune system.

- **Adrenal Gland:** One adrenal gland is attached to the top of each kidney. It produces **adrenaline** and is responsible for the fight-or-flight reactions in the face of danger or stress. The hormones epinephrine and norepinephrine cooperate to regulate states of arousal.

- **Pancreas:** The pancreas is an organ that has both endocrine and exocrine functions. The endocrine functions are controlled by the pancreatic **islets of Langerhans**, which are groups of **beta cells** scattered throughout the gland that secrete **insulin** to lower blood sugar levels in the body. Neighboring **alpha cells** secrete **glucagon** to raise blood sugar.

- **Pineal Gland:** The pineal gland secretes **melatonin**, a hormone derived from the neurotransmitter serotonin. Melatonin can slow the maturation of sperm, oocytes, and reproductive organs. It also regulates the body's **circadian rhythm**, which is the natural awake/asleep cycle. It also serves an important role in protecting the CNS tissues from neural toxins.

- **Testes and Ovaries:** These glands secrete testosterone and estrogen, respectively, and are responsible for secondary sex characteristics, as well as reproduction.

Immune System Structure and Function

The **immune system** is the body's defense against invading microorganisms (bacteria, viruses, fungi, and parasites) and other harmful, foreign substances. It is capable of limiting or preventing infection.

There are two general types of immunity: innate immunity and acquired immunity. **Innate immunity** uses physical and chemical barriers to block the entry of microorganisms into the body. The skin forms a physical barrier that blocks microorganisms from entering underlying tissues. Mucous membranes in the digestive, respiratory, and urinary systems secrete mucus to block and remove invading microorganisms. Saliva, tears, and stomach acids are examples of chemical barriers intended to block infection with microorganisms. In addition, macrophages and other white blood cells can recognize and eliminate foreign objects through phagocytosis or direct lysis.

Acquired immunity refers to a specific set of events used by the body to fight a particular infection. Essentially, the body accumulates and stores information about the nature of an invading microorganism. As a result, the body can mount a specific attack that is much more effective than innate immunity. It also provides a way for the body to prevent future infections by the same microorganism.

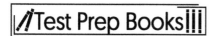

Acquired immunity is divided into a primary response and a secondary response. The **primary immune response** occurs the first time a particular microorganism enters the body, where **macrophages** engulf the microorganism and travel to the lymph nodes. In the lymph nodes, macrophages present the invader to **helper T lymphocytes**, which then activate humoral and cellular immunity. **Humoral immunity** refers to immunity resulting from antibody production by **B lymphocytes**. After being activated by helper T lymphocytes, B lymphocytes multiply and divide into plasma cells and memory cells. Plasma cells are B lymphocytes that produce immune proteins called **antibodies**, or **immunoglobulins**. Antibodies then bind the microorganism to flag it for destruction by other white blood cells. **Cellular immunity** refers to the immune response coordinated by T lymphocytes. After being activated by helper T lymphocytes, other T lymphocytes attack and kill cells that cause infection or disease.

The **secondary immune response** takes place during subsequent encounters with a known microorganism. **Memory cells** respond to the previously encountered microorganism by immediately producing antibodies. Memory cells are B lymphocytes that store information to produce antibodies. The secondary immune response is swift and powerful because it eliminates the need for the time-consuming macrophage activation of the primary immune response. **Suppressor T lymphocytes** also take part to inhibit the immune response as an overactive immune response could cause damage to healthy cells.

Active and Passive Immunity: Immunization is the process of inducing immunity. **Active immunization** refers to immunity gained by exposure to infectious microorganisms or viruses and can be natural or artificial. **Natural immunization** refers to an individual being exposed to an infectious organism as a part of daily life. For example, it was once common for parents to expose their children to childhood diseases such as measles or chicken pox. **Artificial immunization** refers to therapeutic exposure to an infectious organism as a way of protecting an individual from disease. Today, the medical community relies on artificial immunization as a way to induce immunity.

Vaccines are used for the development of active immunity. A **vaccine** contains a killed, weakened, or inactivated microorganism or virus that is administered through injection, by mouth, or by aerosol. Vaccinations are administered to prevent an infectious disease but do not always guarantee immunity.

Passive immunity refers to immunity gained by the introduction of antibodies. This introduction can be natural or artificial. The process occurs when antibodies from the mother's bloodstream are passed on to the bloodstream of the developing fetus. Breast milk can also transmit antibodies to a baby. Babies are born with passive immunity, which provides protection against general infection for approximately the first six months of its life.

Integumentary System (Skin) Structure and Function

Skin consists of three layers: epidermis, dermis, and the hypodermis. There are four types of cells that make up the keratinized stratified squamous epithelium in the epidermis. They are keratinocytes, melanocytes, Merkel cells, and Langerhans cells. Skin is composed of many layers, starting with a basement membrane. On top of that sits the stratum germinativum, the stratum spinosum, the stratum granulosum, the stratum lucidum, and then the stratum corneum at the outer surface. Skin can be classified as thick or thin. These descriptions refer to the epidermis layer. Most of the body is covered with thin skin, but areas such as the palm of the hands are covered with thick skin.

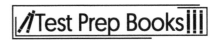

The **dermis** consists of a superficial papillary layer and a deeper reticular layer. The **papillary layer** is made of loose connective tissue, containing capillaries and the axons of sensory neurons. The **reticular layer** is a meshwork of tightly packed irregular connective tissue, containing blood vessels, hair follicles, nerves, sweat glands, and sebaceous glands. The **hypodermis** is a loose layer of fat and connective tissue. Since it is the third layer, if a burn reaches this third degree, it has caused serious damage.

Sweat glands and sebaceous glands are important exocrine glands found in the skin. **Sweat glands** regulate temperature, and remove bodily waste by secreting water, nitrogenous waste, and sodium salts to the surface of the body. Some sweat glands are classified as **apocrine glands**. **Sebaceous glands** are **holocrine glands** that secrete sebum, which is an oily mixture of lipids and proteins. **Sebum** protects the skin from water loss, as well as bacterial and fungal infections.

The three major functions of skin are protection, regulation, and sensation. Skin acts as a barrier and protects the body from mechanical impacts, variations in temperature, microorganisms, and chemicals. It regulates body temperature, peripheral circulation, and fluid balance by secreting sweat. It also contains a large network of nerve cells that relay changes in the external environment to the body.

Lymphatic System Structure and Function

The lymphatic system is one of the major systems that is benefited by proper massage. This system, like the circulatory system, is a network of vessels and organs that move fluid – in this case **lymph** – throughout the body. The lymphatic system works in concert with the immune system, to help the body process toxins and waste. Lymph has a high concentration of white blood cells, which help attack viruses and bacteria throughout body cells and tissues. Lymph is filtered in nodes along the vessels; the body has 600 to 700 lymph nodes, which may be superficial (like those in the armpit and groin) or deep (such as those around the heart and lungs). The **spleen** is the largest organ of the lymphatic system and it helps produce the **lymphocytes** (white blood cells) to control infections. It also controls the number of red blood cells in the body. Other lymphatic organs include the tonsils, adenoids, and thymus.

Muscular System Structure and Function

The muscular system of the human body is responsible for all movement that occurs and the principle system that massage therapists should familiarize themselves with. There are approximately 700 muscles in the body that are attached to the bones of the skeletal system and that make up half of the body's weight. Muscles are attached to the bones through **tendons**. Tendons are made up of dense bands of connective tissue and have collagen fibers that firmly attach to the bone on one side and the muscle on the other. Their fibers are actually woven into the coverings of the bone and muscle so they can withstand the large forces that are put on them when muscles are moving.

There are three types of muscle tissue in the body: **Skeletal muscle** tissue pulls on the bones of the skeleton and causes body movement; **cardiac muscle** tissue helps pump blood through veins and arteries; and **smooth muscle** tissue helps move fluids and solids along the digestive tract and contributes to movement in other body systems. All of these muscle tissues have four important properties in common: They are **excitable,** meaning they respond to stimuli; **contractile,** meaning they can shorten and pull on connective tissue; **extensible**, meaning they can be stretched repeatedly, but maintain the ability to contract; and **elastic**, meaning they rebound to their original length after a contraction.

19

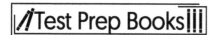

Muscles begin at an **origin** and end at an **insertion**. Generally, the origin is proximal to the insertion and the origin remains stationary while the insertion moves. For example, when bending the elbow and moving the hand up toward the head, the part of the forearm that is closest to the wrist moves and the part closer to the elbow is stationary. Therefore, the muscle in the forearm has an origin at the elbow and an insertion at the wrist.

Body movements occur by muscle contraction. Each contraction causes a specific action. Muscles can be classified into one of three muscle groups based on the action they perform. **Primary movers**, or **agonists**, produce a specific movement, such as flexion of the elbow. **Synergists** are in charge of helping the primary movers complete their specific movements. They can help stabilize the point of origin or provide extra pull near the insertion. Some synergists can aid an agonist in preventing movement at a joint. **Antagonists** are muscles whose actions are the opposite of that of the agonist. If an agonist is contracting during a specific movement, the antagonist is stretched. During flexion of the elbow, the biceps' brachii muscle contracts and acts as an agonist, while the triceps' brachii muscle on the opposite side of the upper arm acts as an antagonist and stretches.

Skeletal muscle tissue has several important functions. It causes movement of the skeleton by pulling on tendons and moving the bones. It maintains body posture through the contraction of specific muscles responsible for the stability of the skeleton. Skeletal muscles help support the weight of internal organs and protect these organs from external injury. They also help to regulate body temperature within a normal range. Muscle contractions require energy and produce heat, which heats the body when cold.

Nervous System Structure and Function

The human nervous system coordinates the body's response to stimuli from inside and outside the body. There are two major types of nervous system cells: neurons and neuroglia. **Neurons** are the workhorses of the nervous system and form a complex communication network that transmits electrical impulses termed **action potentials**, while **neuroglia** connect and support the neurons.

Although some neurons monitor the senses, some control muscles, and some connect the brain to other neurons, all neurons have four common characteristics:

- **Dendrites:** These receive electrical signals from other neurons across small gaps called *synapses*.
- **Nerve cell body:** This is the hub of processing and protein manufacture for the neuron.
- **Axon:** This transmits the signal from the cell body to other neurons.
- **Terminals:** These bridge the neuron to dendrites of other neurons and deliver the signal via chemical messengers called **neurotransmitters.**

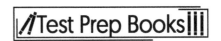

Here is an illustration of a neuron:

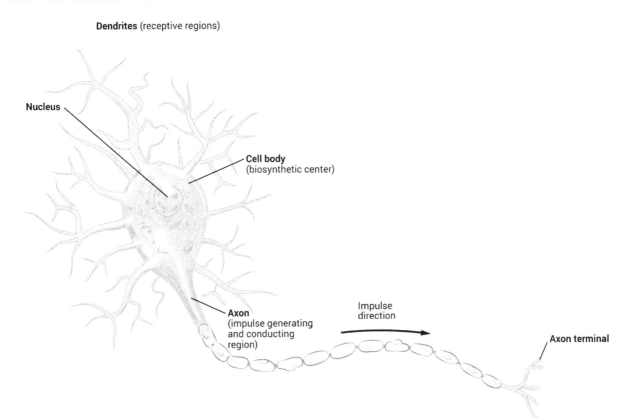

There are two major divisions of the nervous system: central and peripheral.

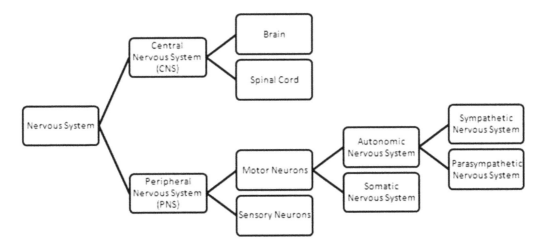

Central Nervous System

The **central nervous system (CNS)** consists of the brain and spinal cord. Three layers of membranes called the **meninges** cover and separate the CNS from the rest of the body.

The major divisions of the brain are the forebrain, the midbrain, and the hindbrain.

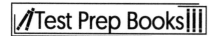
Forebrain

The **forebrain** consists of the cerebrum, the thalamus and hypothalamus, and the rest of the limbic system. The **cerebrum** is the largest part of the brain, and its most well-researched part is the outer cerebral cortex. The cerebrum is divided into right and left hemispheres, and each cerebral cortex hemisphere has four discrete areas, or **lobes**: frontal, temporal, parietal, and occipital. The **frontal lobe** governs duties such as voluntary movement, judgment, problem solving, and planning, while the other lobes are more sensory. The **temporal lobe** integrates hearing and language comprehension, the **parietal lobe** processes sensory input from the skin, and the **occipital lobe** processes visual input from the eyes. For completeness, the other two senses, smell and taste, are processed via the olfactory bulbs. The **thalamus** helps organize and coordinate all of this sensory input in a meaningful way for the brain to interpret.

The **hypothalamus** controls the endocrine system and all of the hormones that govern long-term effects on the body. Each hemisphere of the limbic system includes a **hippocampus** (which plays a vital role in memory), an **amygdala** (which is involved with emotional responses like fear and anger), and other small bodies and nuclei associated with memory and pleasure.

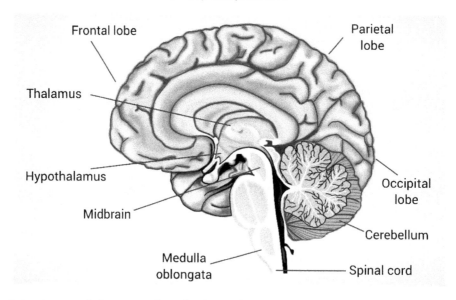

The **midbrain** is in charge of alertness, sleep/wake cycles, and temperature regulation, and it includes the **substantia nigra,** which produces melatonin to regulate sleep patterns. The notable components of the **hindbrain** include the medulla oblongata and cerebellum. The **medulla oblongata** is located just above the spinal cord and is responsible for crucial involuntary functions such as breathing, swallowing, and the regulation of heart rate and blood pressure. Together with other parts of the hindbrain, the midbrain and medulla oblongata form the **brain stem**. The brain stem connects the spinal cord to the rest of the brain. To the rear of the brain stem sits the **cerebellum**, which plays key roles in posture,

22

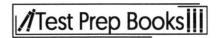

balance, and muscular coordination. The **spinal cord** itself, which is encapsulated by its protective bony **spinal column,** carries sensory information to the brain and motor information to the body.

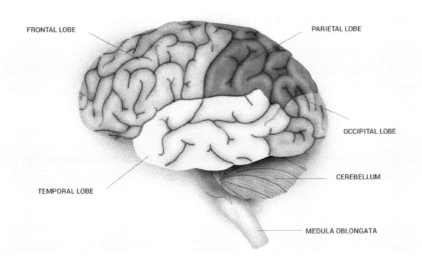

Peripheral Nervous System
The **peripheral nervous system (PNS)** includes all nervous tissue besides the brain and spinal cord. The PNS consists of the sets of cranial and spinal nerves and relays information between the CNS and the rest of the body. The PNS has two divisions: the autonomic nervous system and the somatic nervous system.

Autonomic Nervous System
The **autonomic nervous system (ANS)** governs involuntary, or reflexive, body functions. Ultimately, the autonomic nervous system controls functions such as breathing, heart rate, digestion, body temperature, and blood pressure.

The ANS is split between parasympathetic nerves and sympathetic nerves. These two nerve types are **antagonistic**, and have opposite effects on the body. Parasympathetic nerves predominate resting conditions, and decrease heart rate, decrease breathing rate, prepare digestion, and allow urination and excretion. **Sympathetic nerv**es, on the other hand, become active when a person is under stress or excited, and they increase heart rate, increase breathing rates, and inhibit digestion, urination, and excretion.

Somatic Nervous System and the Reflex Arc
The **somatic nervous system (SNS)** governs the conscious, or voluntary, control of skeletal muscles and their corresponding body movements. The SNS contains afferent and efferent neurons. **Afferent neurons** carry sensory messages from the skeletal muscles, skin, or sensory organs to the CNS. **Efferent neurons** relay motor messages from the CNS to skeletal muscles, skin, or sensory organs.

The SNS also has a role in involuntary movements called **reflexes.** A reflex is defined as an involuntary response to a stimulus. They are transmitted via what is termed a **reflex arc**, where a stimulus is sensed by a receptor and its afferent neuron, interpreted and rerouted by an **interneuron**, and delivered to effector muscles by an efferent neuron where they respond to the initial stimulus. A reflex is able to bypass the brain by being rerouted through the spinal cord; the interneuron decides the proper course

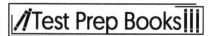

of action rather than the brain. The reflex arc results in an instantaneous, involuntary response. For example, a physician tapping on the knee produces an involuntary knee jerk referred to as the **patellar tendon reflex.**

Reproductive System Structure and Function

The reproductive system is responsible for producing, storing, nourishing, and transporting functional reproductive cells, or gametes, in the human body. It includes the reproductive organs, also known as gonads, the reproductive tract, the accessory glands and organs that secrete fluids into the reproductive tract, and the perineal structures, which are the external genitalia.

The Male System

The male gonads are called **testes**. The testes secrete **androgens**, mainly testosterone, and produce and store 500 million **spermatocytes**, which are the male **gametes**, each day. An androgen is a steroid hormone that controls the development and maintenance of male characteristics. Once the sperm are mature, they move through a duct system, where they mix with additional fluids secreted by accessory glands, forming a mixture called **semen.**

The Female System

The female gonads are the **ovaries**. Ovaries generally produce one immature gamete, an **egg** or **oocyte**, per month. They are also responsible for secreting the hormones estrogen and progesterone. When the oocyte is released from the ovary, it travels along the uterine tubes, or **Fallopian tubes**, and then into the uterus. The **uterus** opens into the **vagina**. When sperm cells enter the vagina, they swim through the uterus and may fertilize the oocyte in the Fallopian tubes. The resulting **zygote** travels down the tube and implants into the uterine wall. The uterus protects and nourishes the developing embryo for nine months until it is ready for the outside environment. If the oocyte is not fertilized, it is released in the uterine, or **menstrual**, cycle. The menstrual cycle occurs monthly and involves the shedding of the functional part of the uterine lining.

Human Reproduction

Humans procreate through sexual reproduction. **Sexual reproduction** involves the fusion of gametes, one from each parent. A **gamete** is a reproductive cell that contains half the chromosomes of a normal cell. Chromosomes are found in the nucleus of cells and contain DNA. The female gamete is called an **ovum**, or **egg**, and the male gamete is called a **sperm**. In sexual reproduction, the gametes fuse through a process called **fertilization**. As a result, sexual reproduction often produces offspring with varying characteristics.

Gametes are created by the human reproductive systems. In women, the ovaries produce eggs, the female gamete. The ovaries produce on average one mature egg per month, which is referred to as the **menstrual cycle**. The release of an egg from the ovaries is termed **ovulation**. The female menstrual cycle is under the control of hormones such as luteinizing hormone (LH), follicle stimulating hormone (FSH), estrogen, and progesterone. In men, the testes produce **sperm**, the male gamete, and they produce millions of sperm at a time. The hormones LH and testosterone regulate the production of sperm in the testes. **Leydig cells** in the testes produce **testosterone,** while sperm is manufactured in the **seminiferous tubules** of the testes.

The fusion of the gametes (egg and sperm) is termed **fertilization**, and the resulting fusion creates a **zygote**. The zygote takes approximately seven days to travel through the fallopian tube and implant

24

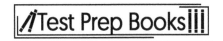

itself into the uterus. Upon implantation, it has developed into a **blastocyst** and will next grow into a **gastrula**. It is during this stage that the embryological germ layers are formed. The three germ layers are the **ectoderm** (outer layer), **mesoderm** (middle layer), and **endoderm** (inner layer). All of the human body systems develop from one or more of the germ layers. The gastrula further develops into an **embryo** which then matures into a **fetus.** The entire process takes approximately nine months and culminates in labor and birth.

Respiratory System Structure and Function

The respiratory system mediates the exchange of gas between the air and the blood, mainly through the act of breathing. This system is divided into the upper respiratory system and the lower respiratory system. The **upper respiratory system** comprises the nose, the nasal cavity and sinuses, and the pharynx. The **lower respiratory system** comprises the **larynx** (voice box), the **trachea** (windpipe), the small passageways leading to the lungs, and the lungs. The upper respiratory system is responsible for filtering, warming, and humidifying the air that gets passed to the lower respiratory system, protecting the lower respiratory system's more delicate tissue surfaces. The process of breathing in is referred to as **inspiration** while the process of breathing out is referred to as **expiration**.

The Lungs

Bronchi are tubes that lead from the trachea to each lung and are lined with cilia and mucus that collect dust and germs along the way. The bronchi, which carry air into the lungs, branch into **bronchioles** and continue to divide into smaller and smaller passageways, until they become **alveoli,** which are the smallest passages. Most of the gas exchange in the lungs occurs between the blood-filled pulmonary capillaries and the air-filled alveoli. Within the lungs, oxygen and carbon dioxide are exchanged between the air in the alveoli and the blood in the pulmonary capillaries. Oxygen-rich blood returns to the heart and is pumped through the systemic circuit. Carbon dioxide-rich air is exhaled from the body. Together, the lungs contain approximately 1,500 miles of airway passages, and this extremely high amount is due to the enormous amount of branching.

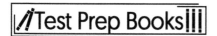
Breathing is possible due to the muscular **diaphragm** pulling on the lungs, increasing their volume and decreasing their pressure. Air flows from the external high-pressure system to the low-pressure system inside the lungs. When breathing out, the diaphragm releases its pressure difference, decreases the lung volume, and forces the stale air back out.

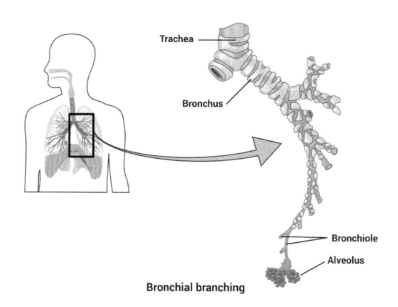

Trachea

Bronchus

Bronchiole

Alveolus

Bronchial branching

Functions of the Respiratory System

The respiratory system has many functions. Most importantly, it provides a large area for gas exchange between the air and the circulating blood. It protects the delicate respiratory surfaces from environmental variations and defends them against pathogens. It is responsible for producing the sounds that the body makes for speaking and singing, as well as for non-verbal communication. It also helps regulate blood volume and blood pressure by releasing vasopressin, and it is a regulator of blood pH due to its control over carbon dioxide release, as the aqueous form of carbon dioxide is the chief buffering agent in blood.

Skeletal System Structure and Function

The **skeletal system** consists of the 206 bones that make up the skeleton, as well as the cartilage, ligaments, and other connective tissues that stabilize them. **Bone** is made of collagen fibers and calcium inorganic minerals, mostly in the form of hydroxyapatite, calcium carbonate, and phosphate salts. The inorganic minerals are strong but brittle, and the collagen fibers are weak but flexible, so the combination makes bone resistant to shattering. There are two types of bone: compact and spongy. **Compact bone** has a basic functional unit, called the **Haversian system**. **Osteocytes**, or bone cells, are arranged in concentric circles around a central canal, called the **Haversian canal**, which contains blood vessels. While Haversian canals run parallel to the surface of the bone, perforating canals, also known as the **canals of Volkmann**, run perpendicularly between the central canal and the surface of the bone.

The concentric circles of bone tissue that surround the central canal within the Haversian system are called **lamellae**. The spaces that are found between the lamellae are called **lacunae**. The Haversian system is a reservoir for calcium and phosphorus for blood. **Spongy bone**, in contrast to compact bone,

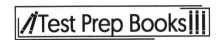

is lightweight and porous. It has a branching network of parallel lamellae, called **trabeculae**. Although spongy bone forms an open framework inside the compact bone, it is still quite strong. Different bones have different ratios of compact-to-spongy bone, depending on their functions. The outside of the bone is covered by a **periosteum**, which has four major functions:

Isolates and protects bones from the surrounding tissue
Provides a place for attachment of the circulatory and nervous system structures
Participates in growth and repair of the bone
Attaches the bone to the deep fascia

An **endosteum** is found inside the bone; it covers the trabeculae of the spongy bone and lines the inner surfaces of the central canals.

One major function of the skeletal system is to provide structural support for the entire body. It provides a framework for the soft tissues and organs to attach to. The skeletal system also provides a reserve of important nutrients, such as calcium and lipids. Normal concentrations of calcium and phosphate in body fluids are partly maintained by the calcium salts stored in bone. Lipids that are stored in yellow bone marrow can be used as a source of energy. Yellow bone marrow also produces some white blood cells. Red bone marrow produces red blood cells, most white blood cells, and platelets that circulate in the blood. Certain groups of bones form protective barriers around delicate organs. The ribs, for example, protect the heart and lungs, the skull encloses the brain, and the vertebrae cover the spinal cord.

Special Senses Structure and Function

The **special senses** include vision, hearing and balance, smell, and taste. They are distinguished from general senses in that special senses have **special somatic afferents** and **special visceral afferents**, both a type of nerve fiber relaying information to the CNS, as well as specialized organs devoted to their function. **Touch** is the other sense that is typically discussed, but unlike the special senses, it relays information to the CNS from all over the body and not just one particular organ; **skin**, the largest organ of the body, is the largest contributor to tactile information, but touch receptors also include **mechanoreceptors** (for touch, pressure, and sound), **nociceptors** (for pain), and **thermoreceptors** (for heat). Nociceptors are divided into mechanosensitive nociceptors (mechanical force), mechanothermal nociceptors (mechanical and thermal stimuli), and polymodal nociceptors (chemical, mechanical, and thermal stimuli). Tactile messages are carried via **general somatic afferents** and **general visceral afferents**. Massage therapists should be familiar with the various touch receptors such as the following:

- **Pacinian corpuscles:** detect rapid vibration in the skin and fascia
- **Meissner's corpuscles:** respond to light touch and slower vibrations
- **Merkel's discs:** respond to sustained pressure
- **Ruffini endings:** detect deep touch and tension in the skin and fascia

Urinary System Structure and Function

The **urinary system** includes the kidneys, ureters, urinary bladder, and the urethra. It is the main system responsible for getting rid of the organic waste products, excess water, and excess electrolytes. The **kidneys** are responsible for producing **urine**, which is a fluid waste product containing water, ions, and small soluble compounds. The urinary system has many important functions related to waste excretion.

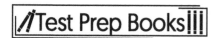

It regulates the concentrations of sodium, potassium, chloride, calcium, and other ions in the plasma by controlling the amount of each that is excreted in urine. This also contributes to the maintenance of blood pH. It regulates blood volume and pressure by controlling the amount of water lost in the urine. It eliminates toxic substances, drugs, and organic waste products, such as urea and uric acid.

The Kidneys

Under normal circumstances, humans have two functioning kidneys. They are the main organs responsible for filtering waste products out of the blood and transferring them to urine. Kidneys are made of millions of tiny filtering units called **nephrons**. Nephrons have two parts: a **glomerulus**, which is the filter, and a **tubule**. As blood enters the kidneys, the glomerulus allows fluid and waste products to pass through it and enter the tubule. Blood cells and large molecules, such as proteins, do not pass through and remain in the blood. The filtered fluid and waste then pass through the tubule, where any final essential minerals are sent back to the bloodstream. The final product at the end of the tubule is **urine**.

Waste Excretion

Once urine accumulates, it leaves the kidneys. The urine travels through the **ureters** into the urinary **bladder**, a muscular organ that is hollow and elastic. As more urine enters the urinary bladder, its walls stretch and become thinner, so there is no significant difference in internal pressure. The urinary bladder stores the urine until the body is ready for urination, at which time the muscles contract and force the urine through the urethra and out of the body.

Tissue Injury and Repair

Healing tissue injuries is a complicated process, mediated by specialized cells. The immune system initiates the response and sends out **macrophages**, which are white blood cells that scavenge for damaged cells and foreign particles. **Fibroblasts** help repair injured cells, laying down **scar tissue**, which is fibrous connective tissue that forms over the injured area. It is denser than healthy tissue. Vitamin C is necessary for tissue repair and Vitamin K plays an instrumental role in blood clotting during initial injury.

Immediately after the injury, there is often bleeding and swelling. The first phase of healing is called the **inflammatory stage**. It takes place from two to three days post-injury to two to three weeks, depending on the injury and the health status of the individual. Bleeding stops during this time and the tissue swells, as the immune system mobilizes the macrophages to the area to clean up debris and prevent infection if the area is open. During the **repair and regeneration phase**, the fibroblasts begin to organize around the site of injury and create new tissue. This occurs anywhere from two to three days to six weeks after the initial injury. After this point and up to a year or so later, the **remodeling phase** occurs, where the scar tissue forms fully over the site of injury.

Concepts of Energetic Anatomy

Massage therapists should familiarize themselves with traditional massage teachings that have an Eastern influence. Regardless of your thoughts on the subject, the concepts of energetic anatomy are increasingly adopted and incorporated into Western massage techniques, and you may be tested on them. Some hold dearly to these methods, but the concepts of energetic anatomy are generally considered pseudoscience.

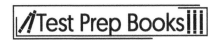

The **Five Elements** is a method based on the ancient Chinese calendar that draws relationships between natural elements, seasons, and body parts. The five elements describe different types of energy. The belief is that massaging the particular body parts associated with the element can increase the emotions and thoughts associated with that element. **Metal** is related to the lungs and large intestine; **Earth** to the spleen and stomach; **fire** is connected with the heart, small intestine, pericardium, and triple heater; **water** to the kidneys and bladder; and **wood**, to the liver and gallbladder. In Indian and Hindu cultures, the term **chakras** is used, which are thought to be the central places in the body that facilitate energy flow. These are also thought of as the seven centers of the **prana**— another word for energy. Thus, these parts of the body are often incorporated in healing methods.

The belief is that **Qi** (also spelled **Chi**) is life energy that continuously flows through the body in pathways called meridians. Interruptions in flow are thought to indicate imbalances in the body and if energy is low, qi flow is believed to be inadequate due to poor organ or tissue function. For therapists using these methods, the goal of massage is to heal the meridians in order to reestablish healthy qi flow, balance, and vitality. This type of therapy is called **Polarity Therapy**. **Meridians** are thought to be in two categories of **yin** and **yang**, with yin meridians flowing upwards and yang meridians flowing downwards. Energetic anatomy identifies twelve principle meridians, with each corresponding to organs of the body.

Levels of Organization of the Human Body

All the parts of the human body are built of individual units called **cells**. Groups of similar cells are arranged into **tissues**, different tissues are arranged into **organs**, and organs working together form entire **organ systems**. The human body has twelve organ systems that govern circulation, digestion, immunity, hormones, movement, support, coordination, urination & excretion, reproduction (male and female), respiration, and general protection.

Body Cavities

The body is partitioned into different hollow spaces that house organs. The human body contains the following cavities:

- **Cranial cavity:** The cranial cavity is surrounded by the skull and contains organs such as the brain and pituitary gland.

- **Thoracic cavity:** The thoracic cavity is encircled by the **sternum** (breastbone) and ribs. It contains organs such as the lungs, heart, **trachea** (windpipe), esophagus, and bronchial tubes.

- **Abdominal cavity:** The abdominal cavity is separated from the thoracic cavity by the diaphragm. It contains organs such as the stomach, gallbladder, liver, small intestines, and large intestines. The abdominal organs are held in place by a membrane called the **peritoneum**.

- **Pelvic cavity:** The pelvic cavity is enclosed by the pelvis, or bones of the hip. It contains organs such as the urinary bladder, urethra, ureters, anus, and rectum. It contains the reproductive organs as well. In females, the pelvic cavity also contains the uterus.

- **Spinal cavity:** The spinal cavity is surrounded by the vertebral column. The vertebral column has five regions: cervical, thoracic, lumbar, sacral, and coccygeal. The spinal cord runs through the middle of the spinal cavity.

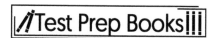

Human Tissues

Human tissues can be grouped into four categories:

Muscle

Muscle tissue supports the body and allows it to move, and muscle cells have the ability to contract. There are three distinct types of muscle tissue: skeletal, smooth, and cardiac. **Skeletal muscle** is voluntary, or under conscious control, and is usually attached to bones. Most body movement is directly caused by the contraction of skeletal muscle. **Smooth muscle** is typically involuntary, or not under conscious control, and it is found in blood vessels, the walls of hollow organs, and the urinary bladder. **Cardiac muscle** is involuntary and found in the heart, which helps pump blood throughout the body.

Nervous

Nervous tissue is unique in that it is able to coordinate information from sensory organs as well as communicate the proper behavioral responses. **Neurons**, or nerve cells, are the workhorses of the nervous system. They communicate via **action potentials** (electrical signals) and **neurotransmitters** (chemical signals).

Epithelial

Epithelial tissue covers the external surfaces of organs and lines many of the body's cavities. Epithelial tissue helps to protect the body from invasion by **microbes** (bacteria, viruses, parasites), fluid loss, and injury. Epithelial cell shapes can be:

- **Squamous:** cells with a flat shape
- **Cuboidal:** cells with a cubed shape
- **Columnar:** cells shaped like a column

Epithelial cells can be arranged in four patterns:

Simple: a type of epithelium composed solely from a single layer of cells

Stratified: a type of epithelium composed of multiple layers of cells

Pseudostratified: a type of epithelium which appears to be stratified but in reality, consists of only one layer of cells

Transitional: a type of epithelium noted for its ability to expand and contract

Connective

Connective tissue supports and connects the tissues and organs of the body. Connective tissue is composed of cells dispersed throughout a **matrix**, which can be gel, liquid, protein fibers, or salts. The primary protein fibers in the matrix are **collagen** (for strength), **elastin** (for flexibility), and **reticulum** (for support). Connective tissue can be categorized as either **loose** or **dense**. Examples of connective tissue include bones, cartilage, ligaments, tendons, blood, and adipose (fat) tissue.

Three Primary Body Planes

A **plane** is an imaginary flat surface. The three primary planes of the human body are frontal, sagittal, and transverse. The **frontal**, or **coronal**, plane is a vertical plane that divides the body or organ into front

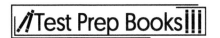
(anterior) and back (posterior) portions. The **sagittal**, or **lateral**, plane is a vertical plane that divides the body or organ into right and left sides. The **transverse plane** is a horizontal plane that divides the body or organ into upper and lower portions.

Like this:

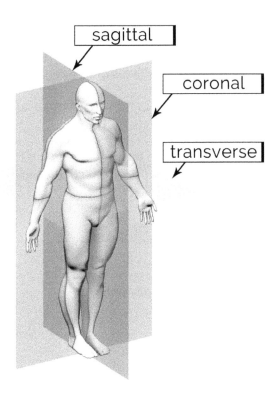

Terms of Direction

- **Medial** refers to a structure being closer to the midline of the body. For example, the nose is medial to the eyes.

- **Lateral** refers to a structure being farther from the midline of the body, and it is the opposite of medial. For example, the eyes are lateral to the nose.

- **Proximal** refers to a structure or body part located near an attachment point. For example, the elbow is proximal to the wrist.

- **Distal** refers to a structure or body part located far from an attachment point, and it is the opposite of proximal. For example, the wrist is distal to the elbow.

- **Anterior** means toward the front in humans. For example, the lips are anterior to the teeth. The term ventral can be used in place of anterior and refers to the abdominal region, or underside, of an organism.

31

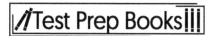

- **Posterior** means toward the back in humans, and it is the opposite of anterior. For example, the teeth are posterior to the lips. The term dorsal can be used in place of posterior and refers to the back or upper side of an organism.

- **Superior** means above and refers to a structure closer to the head. For example, the head is superior to the neck. The terms cephalic or cranial may be used in place of superior.

- **Inferior** means below and refers to a structure farther from the head, and it is the opposite of superior. For example, the neck is inferior to the head. The term caudal may be used in place of inferior and refers to a structure near the tail or posterior of the body.

- **Superficial** refers to a structure closer to the surface. For example, the muscles are superficial because they are just beneath the surface of the skin.

- **Deep** refers to a structure farther from the surface, and it is the opposite of superficial. For example, the femur is a deep structure lying beneath the muscles.

Body Regions

Terms for general locations on the body include:

- **Cervical:** relating to the neck
- **Clavicular:** relating to the clavicle, or collarbone
- **Ocular:** relating to the eyes
- **Acromial:** relating to the shoulder
- **Cubital:** relating to the elbow
- **Brachial:** relating to the arm
- **Carpal:** relating to the wrist
- **Thoracic:** relating to the chest
- **Abdominal:** relating to the abdomen
- **Pubic:** relating to the groin
- **Pelvic:** relating to the pelvis, or bones of the hip
- **Femoral:** relating to the femur, or thigh bone
- **Geniculate:** relating to the knee
- **Pedal:** relating to the foot
- **Palmar:** relating to the palm of the hand
- **Plantar:** relating to the sole of the foot

Abdominopelvic Regions and Quadrants

The **abdominopelvic region** may be defined as the combination of the abdominal and the pelvic cavities. The region's upper border is the breasts and its lower border is the groin region.

The region is divided into the following nine sections:

Right hypochondriac: region below the cartilage of the ribs
Epigastric: region above the stomach between the hypochondriac regions
Left hypochondriac: region below the cartilage of the ribs

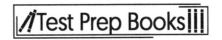

Right lumbar: region of the waist

Umbilical: region between the lumbar regions where the **umbilicus**, or belly button (**navel**), is located

Left lumbar: region of the waist

Right inguinal: region of the groin

Hypogastric: region below the stomach between the inguinal regions

Left inguinal: region of the groin

A simpler way to describe the abdominopelvic area is to divide it into the following quadrants:

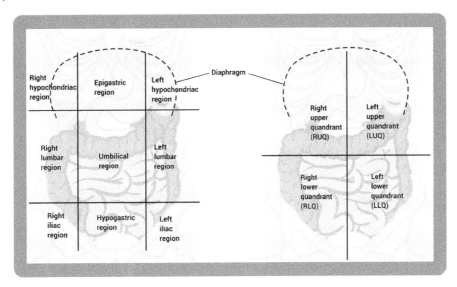

- **Right upper quadrant (RUQ):** Encompasses the right hypochondriac, right lumbar, epigastric, and umbilical regions.

- **Right lower quadrant (RLQ):** Encompasses the right lumbar, right inguinal, hypogastric, and umbilical regions.

- **Left upper quadrant (LUQ):** Encompasses the left hypochondriac, left lumbar, epigastric, and umbilical regions.

- **Left lower quadrant (LLQ):** Encompasses the left lumbar, left inguinal, hypogastric, and umbilical regions.

Kinesiology

Components and Characteristics of Muscles

Muscle anatomy and physiology is rather complex, but it is important for massage therapists to have a solid understanding of the components and characteristics of muscles so that they can provide effective treatment.

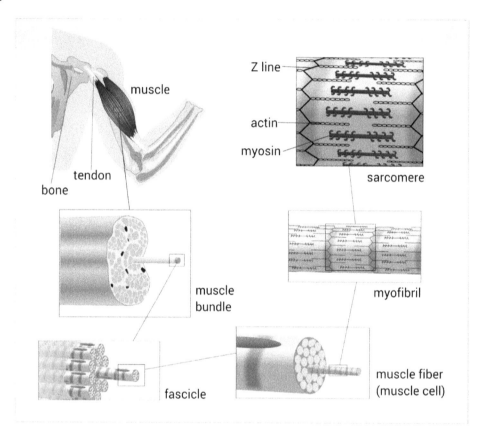

- **Muscle Fibers:** Also called **muscle cells** (i.e., **myocytes**), are long, striated, cylindrical cells that are approximately the diameter of a human hair (50 to 100 um). They have many nuclei dispersed on the outside of the cell and are covered by a fibrous membrane called the **sarcolemma**. Up to 150 muscle fibers can be bundled together into parallel **fasciculi**, with each **fasciculus** being covered by **perimysium** (connective tissue) and each muscle fiber covered by **endomysium.** Each muscle fiber is surrounded by the **sarcolemma** which is a thin, elastic membrane.

- The cytoplasm of a muscle fiber is called the **sarcoplasm**. The sarcoplasm is filled with **myofibrils**, where the components required for muscular contraction exist, including various proteins, protein filaments, mitochondria and the sarcoplasmic reticulum, stored glycogen, enzymes, and fat particles.

34

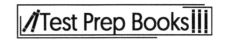

- **Sarcoplasmic reticulum:** A network of tubular channels (called the T-tubule system) and vesicles, which provide structural integrity to the muscle fiber. The sarcoplasmic reticulum also acts as a calcium ion (Ca^{2+}) pump, moving Ca^{2+} ions from the sarcoplasm into the muscle fiber. This influx of Ca^{2+} ions from the sarcoplasm into the muscle fiber results from an action potential in the sarcomere, causing **depolarization**, which initiates muscle movement.

- **Myofibrils:** One of the smaller functional units within a myocyte, consist of long, thin (approximately 1 μm) chains of proteins.

- **Myofilaments:** Primarily consist of chains or filaments of proteins containing actin and myosin. They are the smaller components that make-up the myofibrils within striated muscle fibers.

- **Sarcomere:** The smallest unit of a muscle fiber, contains the actin and myosin proteins responsible for the mechanical process of muscle contractions. Located between two **Z-lines**, the actin and myosin filaments are configured in parallel, end-to-end, along the entire length of the myofibril. The sarcomere consists of four segments: the A-band, H-zone, I-band, and Z-line. The varying arrangement of actin and myosin segments within the sarcomere is responsible for the alternating light and dark pattern of skeletal muscles, producing the striated pattern seen with a microscope. A sarcomere is composed of a basic repeating unit between the Z-lines, located at each end of the sarcomere. The **A-band** contains both actin and myosin. The **H-zone**, a region located in the center of the sarcomere within the A-band, contains only myosin filaments. The **I-band** contains only actin filaments and located by two connected sarcomeres on either side of the Z-line.

- **Transverse-Tubular System:** The T-tubular system is perpendicular to the myofibril and two sarcoplasmic channels. The lateral end of each tubule channel terminates as a **vesicle**, which store calcium. Within each Z-line region, there are two vesicles and a T tubule. The **T tubules** pass through the muscle cell, open externally from the inside of the cell, and touch the sarcolemma on the surface of the cell. The vesicles and T tubules spread the action potential from the surface of the cell's outer membrane almost simultaneously to all inner regions of the cell. This releases the Ca^{2+} from the vesicles, initiating contractile motion.

- **Myosin:** The thick myofilament within a sarcomere, which cross-links with actin filaments. The interaction between these two types of myofilaments causes the sarcomere to shorten as the muscle contracts. Myosin is also responsible for splitting ATP. The phosphate released from ATP hydrolysis into the myosin provides the energy required for the myosin head to produce the power stroke, causing the actin and myosin filaments to slide past each other as muscle contraction occurs. The contraction continues as long as the contraction stimulus and ATP are available.

- **Actin:** A thin myofilament that binds with myosin to cause the sarcomere to contract. Each filament consists of two strands of actin in a double helix configuration. Energy released from ATP hydrolysis generates the power stroke responsible for the actin filaments sliding past the myosin filaments.

- **Troponin:** A protein evenly spaced along the actin filament that binds with Ca^{2+} released from the sarcoplasmic reticulum. The binding of troponin to Ca^{2+} causes a conformational change in tropomyosin, resulting in the binding of the myosin and actin filaments.

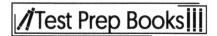

- **Tropomyosin:** A protein in the I-band, which is located along the actin filament in a groove that is formed by the double helix configuration of the two actin strands. The conformational change of troponin moves the tropomyosin deeper into the groove, allowing the actin and myosin cross-bridge to rapidly attach. The actin myofilament is pulled towards the center of sarcomere in a contractile action. When troponin is not affecting tropomyosin (i.e., no Ca^{2+} release), it inhibits actin and myosin from binding, preventing a constant state of muscle contraction.

- **Acetylcholine (ACh):** When an action potential arrives at the terminal end of a motor neuron, vesicles release the neurotransmitter ACh. The ACh diffuses across the synaptic space of the neuromuscular junction, exciting the sarcolemma and starting the process that leads to muscle contraction.

Concepts of Muscle Contraction

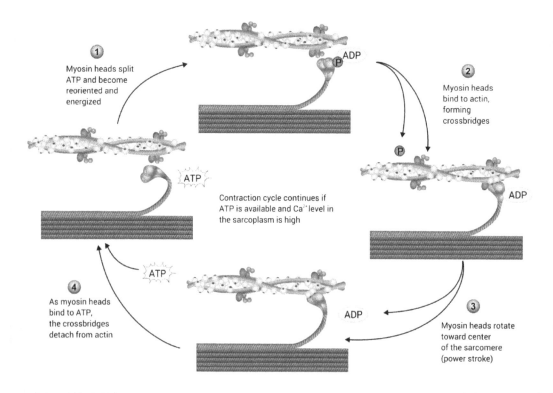

Muscle contraction is explained by the **sliding filament theory**, which states that muscle shortening and lengthening is due to the movement of **actin** (thin filament) and **myosin** (thick filament) sliding past each other. The muscle fiber shortens because the myosin cross-bridges attach, rotate, and detach from actin filaments causing the contractile action. Because minimal calcium is in the myofibril under resting conditions (i.e., during **resting phase**), very few myosin cross-bridges are bound with actin (i.e., actomyosin protein complex). It is during the **excitation-contraction coupling phase** that an electrical discharge at the muscle starts a series of chemical events on the muscle cell surface, resulting in the release of intracellular calcium. The Ca^{2+} binds with troponin, resulting in tropomyosin moving further

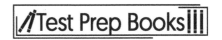

into the double helix groove, allowing rapid binding of actin and myosin filaments and the power stroke that pulls the actin toward the center of the sarcomere.

For this contraction phase to occur, **adenosine triphosphate (ATP)** is broken down into adenosine diphosphate (ADP) by the enzyme myosin **adenosine triphosphatase (ATPase).** The ADP on the myosin globular head is replaced with ATP, resulting in the myosin detaching from the actin and both filaments returning to their original position. If ATP and Ca^{2+} are still available, the entire contraction process is repeated in the muscle fiber during the **recharge phase.** When Ca^{2+}, ATP, ADP, or ATPase are no longer available, relaxation occurs. The **relaxation phase** can also result when the motor neuron stops releasing acetylcholine, Ca^{2+} goes back into the sarcoplasmic reticulum, and the myosin and actin return to their uncoupled resting phase.

The **all-or-none principle** of muscle contraction states that when an action potential in a motor neuron is released into the sarcolemma of a muscle, the action potential will either elicit activation of all the muscle fibers connected to the motor neuron or no activation of any of the muscle fibers will occur. It is not possible to only stimulate some fibers.

There are different muscle contractions that massage therapists should be aware of:

Concentric Contraction
The contraction force is greater than the resistive force, causing the muscle to shorten. The tension caused by the shortening of the muscle causes the joint to move. When a client is doing biceps curls, the elbow is initially extended. The concentric muscle action of the biceps results in the shortening of the muscle, moving the elbow to a flexed position.

Eccentric Contraction
When an external resistance is greater than muscle force, the muscle develops tension and lengthens. During a biceps curl, the lowering of the weight when moving the arm from a flexed to extended position reflects the lengthening of the muscle resulting from eccentric action.

Isometric Contraction
Isometric contraction results when a muscle generates force and attempts to shorten (i.e., concentric action) but is not able to because the resistive force is greater than the muscle source. In this situation, the action does not cause movement (i.e., external work), but it does generate force. If an athlete is holding on to a fixed bar with extended elbows and attempts a concentric action to shorten the biceps, flexing the elbows and moving the bar upwards, the biceps produce force but movement does not occur (i.e., there is no change in the muscle fiber's length) because the resistance is greater than the force generated by the attempted muscle contraction.

Isokinetic Muscle Action
Isokinetic muscle action results in a dynamic movement performed at a constant velocity. Isokinetic muscle actions do not occur naturally. In order for the muscle movement to occur at a constant velocity, a machine, such as a **dynamometer** (a device that allows movement at a constant velocity regardless of the amount of torque), must be used.

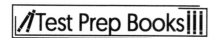

Proprioceptors

Proprioception is one of the main sensory systems of the body. Along with vision, touch, the other special senses, and the vestibular system, **proprioceptors** provide afferent sensory input to the brain about the body and the surroundings. The proprioceptors of the body provide information about the limbs and body as a whole, sensing position, location, orientation, and movement. Proprioception is closely tied with balance and works with the vestibular system to help maintain static position and balance as well as detect when limbs are moving and in what ways. The proprioceptive system has three main goals: to provide awareness of position and kinesthesia within the surroundings, to produce coordinated reflexes to maintain muscle tone and balance, and to provide peripheral feedback information to the central nervous system to help modify movements and motor responses. The body has three types of proprioceptors: muscle spindles, Golgi tendon organs, and joint receptors.

Muscle Spindles

Muscle spindles are proprioceptors located in muscles that sense the rate and magnitude of increasing muscle tension as the muscle lengthens (eccentric muscle contraction). The spindles contain **intrafusal fibers**—modified muscle fibers—that are contained in a sheath of connective tissue and run parallel to the normal **extrafusal muscle fibers**. As a muscle lengthens and stretches, the muscle spindles are also stretched. This activates a **sensory neuron** in the spindle, which sends an impulse to the spinal cord that synapses with the motor neurons, which innervate the extrafusal muscle fibers. The motor neurons activate the muscle, causing a reflexive muscle action—the **stretch reflex**. The muscle contracts, the spindles shorten, and the sensory impulses stop. Increasing loads cause the spindles to stretch more, activating additional muscle force and power, which are potentiated by this reflexive contraction.

Golgi Tendon Organs (GTOs)

Unlike muscle spindles, **GTOs** lie parallel to the extrafusal muscle fibers near the musculotendinous junction and detect changes in the tension of an active muscle. When stimulated, these mechanoreceptors act as feedback monitors and discharge impulses in response to increased tension caused by muscle shortening in order to relax the muscle; this response is also called **autogenic inhibition. Reciprocal inhibition** occurs when a contracting muscle stimulates the GTOs, causing the **antagonist**—opposing—muscle to relax. The GTOs respond to muscle tension by sending impulses to the spinal cord to elicit reflex inhibition. Importantly, GTOs protect the muscle and tendon from injury caused by an excessive load.

Joint Receptors

Joint receptors are found in the capsules and ligaments surrounding the articulations of the skeletal system. Some of these mechanoreceptors are free nerve endings and others are encapsulated within the joints and ligaments. They respond to vibrations, compressions, and tension.

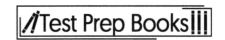

Locations, Attachments, and Actions of Muscles

The following table provides the location, attachments, and actions of the major skeletal muscles organized by body region:

MUSCLE	ORIGIN	INSERTION	ACTION
Sternocleidomastoid	Manubrium of sternum and medial portion of clavicle	Mastoid process, occipital prominence behind the ear	Each muscle pulls head toward opposite shoulder; flexes neck; elevates sternum during rapid breathing
Quadratus lumborum	Iliac crest and lumbar fascia	Transverse processes of upper and lumbar vertebrae and lower margin of 12th rib	Flexes vertebral column laterally, extends lumbar spine (12th rib fixed), assists in forced inspiration
Iliocostalis lumborum	Iliac crest	Lower six ribs	Extends lumbar region of the vertebral column
Iliocostalis thoracis	Lower six ribs	Upper six ribs	Holds spine erect
Iliocostalis cervicis	Upper six ribs	C4-C6 cervical vertebrae	Extends cervical region of the vertebral column
Longissimus thoracis	Transverse processes of lumbar vertebrae	Transverse processes of thoracic and upper lumbar vertebrae and ribs 9 and 10	Extends thoracic region of the vertebral column
Longissimus cervicis	Transverse processes of T4-T5 thoracic vertebrae	Transverse processes of C2-C6 cervical vertebrae	Extends cervical region of the vertebral column
Spinalis thoracis	Spines of upper lumbar and lower thoracic vertebrae	Spines of upper thoracic vertebrae	Extends vertebral column
Spinalis cervicis	Ligamentum nuchae & C7 vertebra	Axis	Extends vertebral column
Spinalis capitis	Spines of upper thoracic and lower cervical vertebrae	Occipital bone	Extends vertebral column

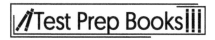

MUSCLE	ORIGIN	INSERTION	ACTION
Trapezius	Occipital bone, ligamentum nuchae, and spines of C7 and all thoracic vertebra	A continuous insertion along acromion and spine of scapula and lateral third of clavicle	Stabilizes, raises, and rotates scapula; middle fibers retract (adduct) scapula; superior fibers elevate scapula (i.e., shrugging shoulders); inferior fibers depress scapula (and shoulder)
Rhomboid major	Spinous processes of T2-T5	Medial (i.e., vertebral) border of scapula	Retracts, elevates, and rotates scapula
Rhomboid minor	Spinous processes of C7-T1	Medial border of scapula	Retracts and elevates scapula
Levator scapulae	Transverse processes of C1-C4	Medial border of scapula	Elevates scapula; flexes neck to same side
Serratus anterior	Series of muscle slips from ribs	Entire anterior (ventral) surface of vertebral border of scapula	Pulls scapula anteriorly and downward; abducts scapula
Pectoralis Minor	Anterior surfaces of ribs 3-5	Coracoid process of scapula	Abducts scapula pulling it forward and downward; draws rib cage superiorly (raises ribs)
Coracobrachialis	Coracoid process of scapula	Medial surface of humerus shaft	Flexes and adducts arm at shoulder; synergist of pectoralis major
Pectoralis Major	Medial ½ of clavicle, sternum, and costal cartilages of ribs 1-6	Greater tubercle of humerus	Prime mover of arm flexion; rotates arm medially, adducts humerus; pulls arm across chest
Teres major	Posterior surface of scapula at inferior angle	Intertubercular groove of the humerus	Postero-medially extends, medially rotates, and adducts humerus; synergist of latissimus dorsi
Latissimus dorsi	Spines of lower six thoracic vertebrae, lumbar vertebrae, lower 3-4 ribs, and iliac crest	Intertubercular groove of the humerus	Prime mover of arm extension; arm adductor; medially rotates humerus at shoulder
Supraspinatus	Supraspinous fossa of scapula	Superior part of greater tubercle of humerus	Assists abduction of arm at shoulder; stabilizes shoulder joint helping to prevent downward dislocation of humerus

40

MUSCLE	ORIGIN	INSERTION	ACTION
Deltoids	Spine of scapula, acromion and lateral 1/3 of clavicle	Deltoid tuberosity of humerus	Prime mover of arm abduction (at shoulder), extends and flexes arm
Subscapularis	Subscapular fossa of scapula	Lesser tubercle of humerus	Medially rotates arm at shoulder
Infraspinatus	Infraspinous fossa of scapula	Greater tubercle of humerus	Laterally rotates arm at shoulder
Teres Minor	Lateral border of dorsal scapular surface	Greater tubercle of humerus	Laterally rotates arm at shoulder
Biceps brachii	Short head: Coracoid process of scapula Long head: Tubercle above glenoid cavity of scapula	Radial tuberosity of radius	Flexes elbow joint and supinates forearm and hand
Brachialis	Anterior, distal ½ of humerus	Coronoid process of the ulna	Flexes elbow
Brachioradialis	Lateral supracondylar ridge at distal end of humerus	Base of styloid process of radius	Flexes forearm at elbow
Triceps brachii	Long Head: Infraglenoid tubercle of scapula Lateral Head: Posterior humerus above radial groove Medial Head: Posterior humerus below	All three heads: Olecranon process of ulna	Extends forearm at elbow
Supinator	Lateral epicondyle of humerus and proximal ulna	Lateral surface of radius	Rotates forearm laterally and supinates hand
Pronator teres	Medial epicondyle of humerus and coronoid process of ulna	Lateral surface of radius	Rotates forearm medially and pronates hand

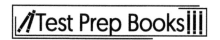

MUSCLE	ORIGIN	INSERTION	ACTION
External oblique	Outer surfaces of lower eight ribs	Outer lip of iliac crest and linea alba	Tenses abdominal wall and compresses abdominal contents
Internal Oblique	Lumbar fascia, iliac crest, and inguinal ligament	Cartilages of lower ribs, linea alba, and crest of pubis	Tenses abdominal wall and compresses abdominal contents
Transverse abdominis	Inguinal ligament, lumbar fascia, cartilages of last 6 ribs, iliac crest	Linea alba and crest of pubis	Compresses abdominal components
Rectus abdominis	Crest of pubis and symphysis pubis	Xiphoid process and costal cartilages of ribs 5-7	Flexes and rotates lumbar region of vertebral column; fixes and depresses ribs, stabilizes pelvis when walking; tenses abdominal wall, increases intra-abdominal pressure
Diaphragm (circular muscle dividing thoracic and abdominal cavities)	Inferior, internal surface of rib cage and sternum, costal cartilages of last six ribs and lumbar vertebrae	Central tendon of diaphragm	Prime mover of inspiration; contraction causes it to flatten out, pulling down lungs for inspiration
External intercostals	Inferior border of rib above	Superior border of rib below	Contraction elevates ribs for inspiration (synergist to diaphragm)
Internal intercostals	Superior border of rib below	Inferior border of rib above	Contraction draws ribs together and depresses rib cage to aid forced expiration
Psoas major (Iliopsoas)	Lumbar intervertebral discs; bodies and transverse processes of lumbar vertebrae	Lesser trochanter of femur via iliopsoas tendon	Flexes thigh; also effects lateral flexion of vertebral column; important postural muscle
Iliacus (Iliopsoas)	Iliac fossa and crest, lateral sacrum	Femur on and immediately below lesser trochanter of femur via iliopsoas tendon	Prime mover for flexing thigh or for flexing trunk on thigh during a bow
Gluteus maximus (Glutes)	Sacrum, coccyx, and posterior surface of ilium	Posterior surface of femur and fascia of thigh	Major extensor of thigh; generally inactive during standing and walking; laterally rotates and abducts thigh

42

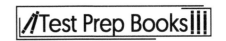

MUSCLE	ORIGIN	INSERTION	ACTION
Gluteus medius	Lateral surface of ilium	Greater trochanter of femur	Abducts and medially rotates thigh; stabilizes pelvis; extremely important in walking
Gluteus minimus	Lateral surface of ilium	Anterior border of greater trochanter of femur	Abducts and rotates thigh medially (same as gluteus medius)
Piriformis	Anterior surface of sacrum	Superior border of greater trochanter of femur	Abducts and rotates thigh laterally; stabilizes hip joint
Tensor fasciae latae	Anterior iliac crest	Iliotibial tract (fascia of thigh)	Abducts, flexes, and rotates thigh medially
Pectineus	Spine of pubis	Femur distal to lesser trochanter	Adducts, flexes, and medially rotates thigh
Adductor brevis	Body and inferior ramus of pubis	Posterior surface of femur	Adducts and medially and laterally rotates thigh
Adductor longus	Pubic bone near symphysis pubis	Posterior surface of femur (linea aspera)	Adducts, flexes, and medially and laterally rotates thigh
Adductor magnus	Ischial tuberosity	Linea aspera and adductor tubercle of femur	Anterior part adducts and medially rotates and flexes thigh; posterior part is a synergist of hamstrings in thigh extension
Gracilis	Lower edge of symphysis pubis	Medial surface of tibia	Adducts thigh, flexes and medially rotates thigh (especially during walking), flexes knees
Sartorius	Anterior superior iliac spine	Medial surface of tibia	Flexes knee and hip, abducts and rotates thigh laterally
Biceps femoris	Ischial tuberosity (long head); linea aspera and distal femur (short head)	Head of fibula and lateral condyle of tibia	Extends thigh and flexes knee; laterally rotates leg, especially when knee is flexed
Semitendinosus	Ischial tuberosity	Medial aspect of upper tibial shaft	Extends thigh at hip; flexes knee; with semimembranosus, medially rotates leg
Semimembranosus	Ischial tuberosity	Medial condyle of tibia	Extends thigh and flexes knee; medially rotates leg
Rectus femoris	Iliac spine and margin of acetabulum	Patella and tibial tuberosity via patellar ligament	Extends knee and flexes thigh at hip

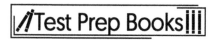

MUSCLE	ORIGIN	INSERTION	ACTION
Vastus lateralis	Greater trochanter, intertrochanteric line, linea aspera	Patellar ligament to tibial tuberosity	Extends and stabilizes knee
Vastus medialis	Linea aspera, intertrochanteric line	Patellar ligament to tibial tuberosity	Extends knee; inferior fibers stabilize patella
Vastus intermedius	Anterior and lateral surfaces of proximal femur shaft	Patellar ligament to tibial tuberosity	Extends knee
Gastrocnemius	Lateral and medial condyles of femur	Posterior surface of calcaneus	Ankle plantarflexion, flexes knee
Soleus	Head and shaft of fibula and posterior surface of tibia	Posterior surface of calcaneus	Ankle plantarflexion
Plantaris	Posterior femur above lateral condyle	Calcaneus	Ankle plantarflexion, flexes knee
Flexor digitorum longus	Posterior surface of tibia	Distal phalanges of four lateral toes	Ankle plantarflexion and inversion of foot, flexes four lateral toes
Tibialis posterior	Lateral condyle and posterior surface of tibia and posterior surface of fibula	Tarsal and metatarsal bones	Ankle plantarflexion and inversion of foot
Fibularis (peroneus) longus	Lateral condyle of tibia and head and shaft of fibula	Tarsal and metatarsal bones	Ankle plantarflexion and eversion of foot, also supports arch
Tibialis anterior	Lateral condyle and lateral surface of tibia	Inferior surface of medial cuneiform and first metatarsal bone	Prime mover of dorsiflexion; inversion of the foot
Fibularis (peroneus) tertius	Distal anterior surface of fibula	Dorsal surface of fifth metatarsal	Prime mover of toe extension; dorsiflexion and eversion of foot
Extensor digitorum longus	Lateral condyle of tibia and anterior surface of fibula	Dorsal surface of second and third phalanges of four lateral toes	Ankle dorsiflexion and eversion of foot, extends toes

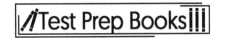

MUSCLE	ORIGIN	INSERTION	ACTION
Extensor hallucis longus	Anteromedial fibula shaft	Distal phalanx of the great toes	Extends great toe, ankle dorsiflexion and inversion of foot

Joint Structure and Function

Joints can be classified based on the structure of how the bones are connected:

- **Fibrous joints:** Bones joined by fibrous tissue and that lack a joint cavity (e.g., sutures of the skull)

- **Cartilaginous joints:** Bones joined by cartilage and that lack a joint cavity (e.g., the pubic symphysis)

- **Synovial joints:** Bones separated by a fluid-containing joint cavity with articular cartilage covering the ends of the bone and forming a capsule

- **Plane joints:** Flat surfaces that allow gliding and transitional movements (e.g., intercarpal joints)

- **Hinge joints:** Cylindrical projection that nests in a trough-shaped structure, single plane of movement (e.g., the elbow)

- **Pivot joints:** Rounded structure that sits into a ring-like shape, allowing uniaxial rotation of the bone around the long axis (e.g., radius head on ulna)

- **Condyloid joints:** Oval articular surface that nests in a complementary depression, allowing all angular movements (e.g., the wrist)

- **Saddle joints:** Articular surfaces that have both complementary concave and convex areas, allowing more movement than condyloid joints (e.g., the thumb)

- **Ball-and-socket joints:** Spherical structure that fits in a cuplike structure, allowing multiaxial movements (e.g., the shoulder)

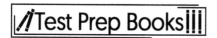

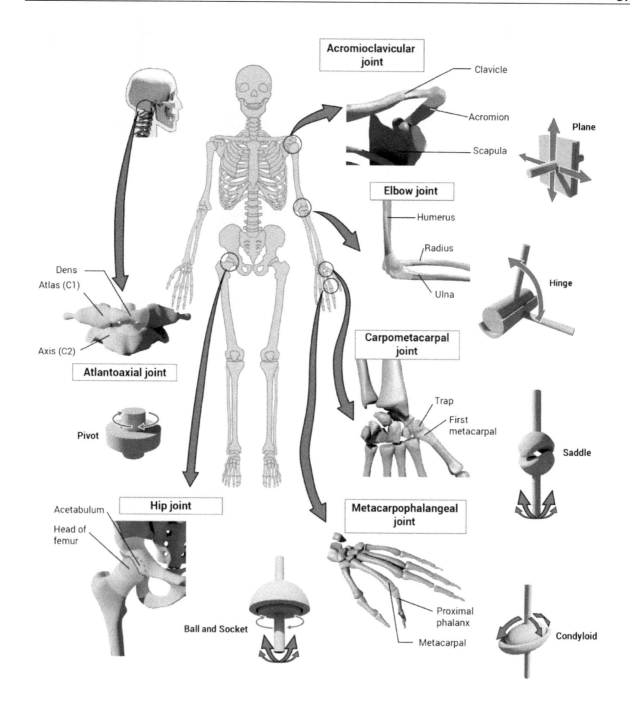

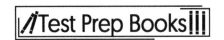
Range of Motion

Range of motion refers to the amount of movement or distance that a joint can travel between the fully flexed and extended positions. Massage therapists and fitness and bodywork professionals use various stretching modalities to try to increase range of motion when it is limited due to tightness in series, elastic, or contractile elements of muscles, tendons, fascia, ligaments, or cartilage surrounding a joint. Inflammation within the joint space can also reduce the available range of motion, as can pain and guarding.

- **Passive range of motion** refers to the motion that the joint allows entirely under the therapist's control; the client remains completely relaxed and allows the therapist to manually move the limb segments around the joint to assess the available motion. Passive range of motion only assesses the non-contractile structures surrounding a joint, and any hypermobility or limited range of motion can be assessed in structures such as ligaments, joint capsules, and fasciae.

- With **active range of motion**, the client uses their muscles to move the joint instead of the therapist providing the mechanical power. In this way, active range of motion assesses both the non-contractile and contractile elements, including the muscles and tendons themselves. If a therapist determines that there is hypomobility at a joint due to the limitations in the contractile components, massage can be useful in bringing blood flow to the area and attempting to break up any adhesions or tightness within the fibers and tissues.

- **Resisted range of motion** is a form of active range of motion testing in which the therapist assesses the strength of the muscles and contractile elements surrounding the joint. The joint is placed in its neutral position. The client is asked to contract the muscles to either flex or extend the joint being evaluated, while the therapist provides resistance in the form of the opposing motion at the joint. For example, when evaluating biceps flexion strength, the arm should be held at the side in the neutral position. Then the client is asked to flex the arm, bending the elbow. The therapist should place their hands on the forearm just above the wrist and just below the shoulder on the upper arm, isolating the elbow joint.

The therapist should be mindful to never cross two joints at once with their hand position, because this can cause injury. While the client flexes their elbow, the therapist provides an extension force to the elbow, countering flexion and providing resistance. The therapist can gauge the strength of the client's contraction based on the amount of resistance he or she can apply to the joint. This type of exercise is contraindicated for any client who has an acute injury to the area being evaluated. The amount of resistance provided by the massage therapist should be appropriate to the health and physical ability of the client; maximal resistance is never recommended.

Pathology, Contraindications, Areas of Caution, Special Populations

Overview of Pathologies

The following are some basic pathologies that clients may experience. Massage therapists should familiarize themselves with these conditions and the impact of massage on them. Certain pathologies are absolute contraindications, or medical reasons for not performing massage therapy. Other conditions can be improved with massage.

Acne: the appearance of many small blisters on any area of the body due to clogged pores or naturally oily skin. Massage directly over the affected area is contraindicated.

Asthma: difficulty breathing, caused by the constriction and inflammation of the bronchial tubes. Massage can decrease overall stress, soothe inflammation, and improve quality of life.

Alzheimer's: a degenerative disease-causing dementia, most common in the elderly. Massage can be helpful in relieving stress, but the therapist should be patient and cautious. If possible, the client's primary caretaker should be present during treatment.

Bone fractures/breaks: a break or crack in bone. Fractures can be classified in several ways: they may be **open** (bone pieces have broken through the skin) or **closed**; **complete** (bone is fractured all the way through) or **incomplete** (a crack such as a stress fracture, hairline fracture, or greenstick fracture); or classified based on the type of fracture, such as spiral, comminuted, longitudinal, etc. Massage is contraindicated on the site of the injury. Gentle effleurage or long, broad strokes applied proximal to the break may help relieve swelling and inflammation.

Burns and open wounds: a tissue injury caused by heat, electricity, friction, radiation, or chemicals that damages some or all layers of the epidermis and dermis. They are classified based on the severity, with **first-degree burns** being contained to more superficial layers of the epidermis to **third-degree burns**, which may extend to damage underlying muscle, bone, nerve, and adipose tissue. Massage is contraindicated over any broken skin; the therapist should never touch blood or pus from a wound.

Cancer: the growth of tumors in one or more areas of the body. Oncology massage is a very specialized modality and should only be performed by a qualified and certified therapist. Depending on the severity of the situation, the therapist may work under the supervision of a doctor.

Carpal tunnel syndrome: paresthesia in the thumb, index and middle fingers, and the medial side of the ring finger, caused by the compression of the median nerve in the carpal tunnel. Massage is indicated and can effectively relieve symptoms.

Cold/flu: viral infections of the upper respiratory tract. Massage is an absolute contraindication in the acute stages of illness, due to contagion and the overproduction of phlegm. Massage in this stage can overwhelm the lymphatic system. In later, less acute stages, gentle massage is indicated.

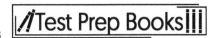
Deep Vein Thrombosis (DVT): a clot located in a vein, usually in the lower extremities. The danger is that the clot will dislodge and circulate to the heart, causing a heart attack. Massage is locally contraindicated.

Depression: a chronic mood disorder involving decreased energy levels and sadness. Massage is indicated and can be a vital part of treatment. Touch stimulates neurochemicals that increase a sense of happiness and well-being, and detailed myofascial release can improve posture and confidence.

Diabetes: a disease in which the body cannot produce enough insulin, the hormone that controls carbohydrate metabolism, or does not effectively use insulin. As a result, diabetics can have irregular blood sugar levels. Diabetes is not contagious, and massage is indicated to relieve stress and improve circulatory issues that are common in diabetics.

Eczema: a congenital skin condition, presenting as red or bumpy areas. Eczema is often found around joints or crevices of the body, such as the elbows or neck. It is not contagious, and specialists believe flare-ups are stress-related. Massage is indicated with the use of hypoallergenic lotion.

Edema: the buildup of fluid in an area of the body, usually a limb. Edema is not in itself dangerous, but it can be a sign of a very serious condition. Light effleurage, proximal to the swelling and with strokes leading back toward the heart, can help alleviate symptoms.

Pitting edema: indicated by the skin retaining an indentation mark after it is pushed, pressed, or pinched. It is a contraindication for massage as it may indicate a cardiovascular or renal issue.

Fever: systemic inflammation, characterized by a body temperature above the normal 98.6 degrees. Massage is strictly contraindicated as it stimulates blood flow, thus increasing the inflammation.

Fibromyalgia: idiopathic body-wide pain. Massage is indicated and may be a primary component of the treatment plan, alleviating symptoms and improving overall wellbeing.

Fungal infections: the overgrowth of fungus in the skin or nails, causing discoloration and a spongy or boggy texture. Massage is contraindicated in the affected area for the safety of the therapist.

Headaches: pain in the head stemming from numerous ailments. Massage is indicated for tension headaches and some migraines. The therapist should check in with the client during the session and immediately cease any techniques that cause a headache to worsen.

Hepatitis: a collection of diseases causing liver dysfunction. Strains of hepatitis are designated by letters: Hep A, Hep B, and Hep C. Massage is indicated as long as standard precautions and hygiene practices are used.

Hernia: a tear in a muscle wall, which can cause organs or other structures to get trapped as the muscle heals. Massage is locally contraindicated.

Herniated disc: the partial or complete displacement of an intervertebral disc, resulting in nerve pain and muscle spasm. Acute or long-term injuries to the spinal column result in herniation of the intervertebral discs. **Discs** are spongy structures, located between each of the vertebrae. They protect the vertebrae and spinal cord and absorb impact as the spine moves.

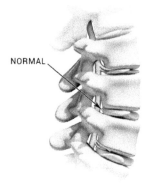
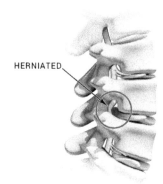

Acute herniation occurs when these discs are twisted or pulled too far in one direction, and herniation can also occur from chronic weakening of the annulus fibrosis surrounding the disc. The inside of the disc, the **nucleus pulposus**, bulges out of the intervertebral joint and can no longer protect the nerves in the spinal cord. The surrounding muscles spasm in order to compensate and protect the injured area, which can be extremely painful. In addition, the nerves emerging from the spinal cord can become irritated and radiate pain along their entire length. This most often presents as cervical nerves causing pain in the upper back (especially rhomboids) and lumbar nerves (most often the sciatic nerve) sending pain down the legs.

Massage is indicated to relieve these symptoms and improve posture, which can help the disc move back into place. When working with clients who suffer from herniated discs, the massage therapist has two goals: (1) to relieve the acute pain and (2) to address the root cause of the disc injury. Tractioning techniques are especially helpful for these clients as the techniques have the dual impact of relieving pressure on the herniated disc (thus allowing it to move back into place in the spine) and also stretching the spasming muscles to relieve pain.

HIV/AIDS: a contagious autoimmune disease, transmitted by the contact of blood, pre-seminal fluids, semen, vaginal fluids, rectal fluids, or breast milk with a mucous membrane or open wound. HIV/AIDS can be deadly, but treatment of the disease has vastly improved in recent years. HIV/AIDS *cannot* be passed by touching skin to skin, unless the skin is broken. Massage is indicated, as long as the therapist does not come into contact with the client's bodily fluids.

Hives: raised, itching red bumps on the skin, usually due to allergic reactions. Massage is contraindicated directly over the swelling, but it is important to note that hives are not contagious.

Hypertension: high blood pressure, often asymptomatic until it results in a heart attack or stroke. Massage is indicated for clients with controlled hypertension, as long as modifications are used. For acute or untreated cases, massage is absolutely contraindicated.

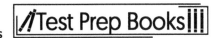
Hyperthyroidism: a condition in which the thyroid produces excessive T3 and T4, resulting in uncontrollable weight loss and elevated body temperature. Massage is indicated.

Hypothyroidism: the inability of the thyroid to produce adequate levels of T3 and T4, resulting in sluggishness and weight gain, among other symptoms. In some patients, this condition can also cause atherosclerosis. Massage is indicated unless atherosclerosis is present.

Inflammation: the presence of four characteristic symptoms: heat, redness, swelling, and pain. A fever, for example, is a kind of inflammation that impacts the entire body. Individual muscles or joints can also become inflamed if they sustain injuries. While painful, inflammation is not always a negative thing; in fact, this process is necessary for healing and muscle growth.

A massage therapist should assess the situation and choose whether to decrease or stimulate inflammation in a particular area. For acute injuries, such as muscle strains or hematomas sustained from impact, decreasing inflammation is important. Ice will help calm down the immediate area, and gentle effleurage and flushing techniques will draw swelling away from the site of injury. For chronic pain—for example, the neck pain of a desk worker—the LMT should instead stimulate inflammation, which reminds the brain of the site of the initial injury, to initiate the healing process. Trigger point therapy, heat packs applied to the site, and deep tissue techniques are helpful in these cases.

Insomnia: the inability to sleep consistently or for long periods of time. Massage is indicated as it stimulates the production of serotonin and induces relaxation. **Serotonin** is necessary for the production of **melatonin**, the neurochemical most important in circadian rhythm and the sleep-wake cycle.

Lupus: a chronic disease in which the immune system attacks the body's own tissues and organs, creating ongoing inflammation. Lupus follows the flare-up/remission pattern of most autoimmune diseases. Massage is contraindicated during flare-ups, but it can help during remissions.

Lice: small mites found in the hair, most often on the scalp or pubis. Lice are extremely contagious; massage is contraindicated until the infection has been treated.

Moles: irregular bumps and birthmarks, often small and round. Massage is indicated unless there is visible broken skin or the client finds it painful to the touch.

Mononucleosis: a virus with flu-like symptoms, especially causing extreme fatigue. Massage is absolutely contraindicated until the client is completely healed, due to the contagious nature of the disease.

Multiple Sclerosis (MS): an autoimmune disease that attacks the myelin that insulates neurons. Clients may experience slow or rapid degeneration of nerve function. Massage is contraindicated during a flare-up, but indicated when the disease is in remission.

Muscle spasms: the involuntary contraction of a muscle due to injury. Muscles go into spasm to protect themselves and the surrounding structures from further damage. Gentle massage is indicated, but the therapist should never completely relieve an acute spasm. More vigorous techniques may be used for chronic muscle spasms.

Osteoarthritis: the inflammation and breakdown of the cartilage in one or more joints. It can be caused by the wear and tear of a long life or by an injury. Massage is indicated for pain relief in the joint itself and compensating muscles.

Osteoporosis: a condition in which bones become thin and brittle from a lack of calcium and vitamin D. Gentle massage is indicated for pain relief. Deep tissue massage is absolutely contraindicated, and the therapist should consult a physician if the client's case is severe.

Plantar fasciitis: the thickening and tightening of the plantar fascia, most often presenting as pain upon standing after a long period of rest. Massage is indicated, especially deep friction techniques, to break up the scar tissue.

Premenstrual syndrome (PMS): pain and hormonal changes immediately preceding the menses. Massage is indicated and can help relieve symptoms.

Psoriasis: a congenital condition presenting as the thickening and flaking of the skin, characterized by a scaly, dry appearance. Massage is indicated and can help alleviate symptoms.

Renal failure: the degeneration and failure of the kidneys. Massage is absolutely contraindicated as it increases circulation of blood and lymph and can place undue stress on the body.

Rheumatoid Arthritis: an autoimmune condition in which the joint capsule is attacked, causing pain and degeneration of ligament and even bone. Gentle massage and myofascial release are indicated.

Scar tissue: connective tissue that forms at the site after an injury. Its composition varies depending on how recently it has formed. Newly formed scar tissue is composed primarily by fibroblasts, while older scar tissue is mainly dense collagenous fibers. Even invisible scars can have a systemic impact on fascia. Massage is indicated to relieve tightness that results from irregular scar tissue, and friction techniques can be used to break up and heal the scar itself.

Shin splints: an umbrella term for a collection of anterior leg injuries, including tendinitis and muscle spasms. Massage is indicated and should be combined with stretching or physical therapy.

Strains and sprains: Strains and sprains, while mechanically similar, are two different kinds of injuries. **Strains** occur when a muscle or tendon is damaged, while **sprains** involve damage to a ligament. Strains and sprains are both classified as either Grade I, II, or III:

- **Grade I injuries** include minor tearing or overstretching of the involved structures, resulting in pain and inflammation.

- **Grade II injuries** are more severe and include partial tearing of the muscle or ligament. This can cause severe pain and take much longer to heal than a Grade I injury.

- **Grade III injuries**, the most severe, involve a complete tear or rupture. For strains, this means the muscle is torn through and has detached from one of its insertions. This usually presents as a large bulge in the area where the torn muscle has bunched up, since it is no longer stretched along a bone. In a Grade III sprain, one or more ligaments snap like a rubber band that has been stretched too tight.

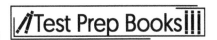
Treatment for these injuries varies depending on their severity. The body can heal many of these injuries through the inflammation process, where blood flow is increased to the area. For more severe injuries, medical intervention is required and can range from treatments such as injections to physical therapy to surgery.

Stroke: the temporary interruption of blood flow to some or all of the brain, often caused by clotting. Massage is indicated for some stroke sufferers, as long as the therapist is in close communication with the client's physician.

Tendinitis: inflammation of the tendon or tendinous sheath of a particular muscle due to injury or overuse, presenting with chronic pain and/or weakness. Massage is indicated only if specific protocols are used to break up any scar tissue, control inflammation, and stimulate the fascial regeneration.

Temporomandibular Joint Dysfunction (TMJD): any one of a collection of disorders affecting the temporomandibular joint. TMJD is often caused by tooth-grinding and can result in severe headaches. Intraoral massage and trigger point therapy are indicated.

Ulcers: sores that do not heal, caused by pressure or inflammation. Ulcers are found anywhere in or on the body. Massage is locally contraindicated for ulcers on the skin. Gentle techniques, like light effleurage or craniosacral therapy, can help improve some stomach ulcers.

Varicose veins: visibly distended or dark-colored veins, usually in the legs. Deep pressure is contraindicated over the site; light, brief effleurage is not harmful.

Warts: localized skin lesions, rough and discolored in appearance, caused by the human papillomavirus (HPV). Warts are contagious, and massage is locally contraindicated.

Contraindications

Contraindications are existing conditions that prevent a client from safely and healthily receiving massage.

Absolute contraindications mean that the client should not receive massage at all until the issue is resolved. Examples of absolute contraindications include fevers and infectious diseases, acute hypertension, shock, and recent trauma, such as a car accident.

Regional contraindications make it safe for clients to receive massage on parts of their bodies that are unaffected. Broken skin due to burns or open wounds, broken bones, and varicose veins are examples of regional contraindications.

It is vital that the massage therapist get a detailed and thorough medical history from each client before performing massage in order to respect any contraindications that may be present.

Infections
Infections are defined as the harmful microbes causing localized or systemic damage to the body. Bacterial infections are treated with antibiotics, which are extremely effective but have the side effect of destroying helpful bacteria, especially the flora in the digestive system. When working with a client who has an infection, the massage therapist should get as much information as he or she can about its

progression. Performing massage on a client who has an untreated infection can be dangerous for both the client and the therapist.

Cold/Flu Symptoms

Acute cold and flu symptoms are an absolute contraindication to massage. If a client is no longer contagious, but continues to cough or sneeze as they flush out phlegm from their system, the massage therapist should use their best judgment; often, massage can be helpful to break up and flush out the phlegm. However, working with someone that is still contagious can be dangerous to both the client and the therapist. For one thing, the massage therapist will put himself/herself and all other clients at risk of contagion.

Also important is the negative impact on the sick client's health. Massage increases circulation and can make lymph move through the system more quickly. This has the effect of spreading sickness throughout the body and overwhelming the immune system, making it harder for the client to fight off infection or heal from a disease he or she already has. Moreover, this process diminishes any other positive effects of massage as it makes the muscles unnecessarily sore and sensitive. When faced with the option of treating a client who has acute, contagious flu symptoms, a massage therapist should decline treatment until the symptoms subside.

Site Specific Contraindications

Site-specific contraindications mean the therapist should avoid working directly on the affected area, although massage on the rest of the body is fine. Broken bones, contagious or painful skin conditions, and fungal infections are examples of site-specific contraindications.

Skin Conditions

Massage therapists are in a unique position to see many kinds of skin conditions on their clients. It is important to have some knowledge about the differences between these conditions.

- **Eczema** is the thickening and flaking of the skin and is characterized by a scaly, dry appearance. Eczema is not dangerous or contagious and can benefit from the application of hypoallergenic lotion to the affected area.

- **Hives** and **bug bites** are visually similar. Usually, they appear as a small raised red bump, surrounded by a few inches of red or swollen skin. Neither of these are contagious, but if a client has scratched the area, there may be broken skin. Hives are not to be confused with poison ivy or poison oak, both of which are highly contagious and painful. A client with a raised, regular rash that has no discernible site of injury (i.e., a central bug bite or hive) may be suffering from a run-in with one of these plants. These rashes represent a local contraindication.

- **Acne** is a more common and more persistent skin irritation. While not contagious on its own, it can indicate a high risk of broken skin, which can be dangerous for the massage therapist. It can also be painful for a client to receive pressure on the skin in the middle of a break-out. When working with a client who has this condition, it is best to check with him or her before using any lotion or oil as some chemicals can further irritate the skin.

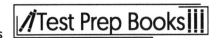

- Most discoloration of the skin can be attributed to rashes, moles, or birthmarks, but can also indicate skin cancer. Many massage therapists are credited with saving clients' lives by discovering cancerous moles in locations no one else would see, such as the middle of the back or the posterior thigh. Always remember the **ABCDE of skin cancer:**

  o Cancer moles are **A**symmetrical.
  o They present irregular **B**orders.
  o They contain abnormal **C**olors, or multiple colors, in one mole.
  o They have a **D**iameter of more than ¼ inch.
  o Cancer moles **E**volve or change over time.

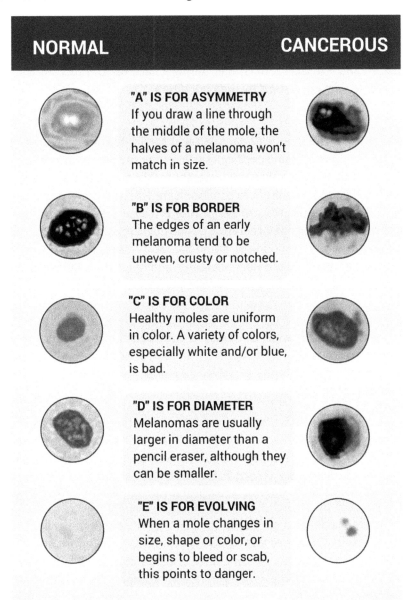

If a therapist believes a client may have a cancerous mole, it is always better to mention it. Potentially saving someone's life is a lot more important than avoiding an awkward or difficult conversation.

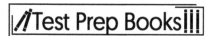

Fungal Infections

Fungal infections are extremely common, affecting an estimated 25% of the population worldwide. Some forms of fungus are more contagious than others. For example, infections of the fingernails and toenails are highly contagious and difficult to cure. These infections are characterized by spongy or discolored nails; most often the nail will be abnormally thick and textured and appear yellow or black. Fungal infections can also occur in the skin, feeding off cutaneous tissue. These can be recognized by discoloration and circular, sometimes ring-like, patterns. A massage therapist should use their judgment when deciding whether to work with a client who exhibits signs of fungal infection. While technically risky—especially in cases affecting the nails—infections of this kind do not always transmit from person to person and do not always present symptoms.

Pathology-Related Contraindications

Modifications are sometimes necessary for clients with chronic illnesses. Clients with autoimmune diseases, for example, should not receive massages during a flare-up. During remission, however, bodywork can help reverse damage caused by their condition.

Multiple Sclerosis

MS is an autoimmune disease. The immune system attacks the body, breaking down vital systems over time. In this disease, the immune system specifically attacks the myelin sheaths of neurons. As a result, the electrical impulses sent by the nervous system are not insulated when they travel down the axon of a neuron. This makes it difficult for the brain to communicate with the body, and patients experience a loss of muscle control. In severe cases, MS can even cause brain damage and cognitive dysfunction. In some cases, damaged myelin can regenerate during periods of remission. Massage can be especially helpful in these cases as it promotes blood flow, stimulates and relaxes muscles that experience **paresthesia** (or "pins and needles") due to nerve damage, and helps the client relax and focus on the healing process.

Cancer

The question of offering massage to cancer patients is a controversial one. Until very recently, it was believed that massage would cause cancer to spread from one area of the body to another. However, research shows that stimulating the lymphatic system and inducing relaxation with massage techniques can improve the symptoms of this disease.

Oncology massage is a specific modality that provides vital education to therapists and enables them to provide healthy and helpful care to these special clients. It is important that therapists working with cancer clients be certified in oncology massage. In some cases, they may work directly with a client's medical team, but this is not mandatory as long as the therapist obtains a very thorough history from the client. Any questions should be directed to a medical professional.

The therapist should be knowledgeable about the specific type of cancer their client suffers from. **Leukemia**, for example, affects the bones and blood and, therefore, the entire body. Other forms of cancer are extremely localized; in these cases, massage is locally contraindicated over the site of the tumor. In the case of clients who undergo surgery to remove tumors, the incision site represents another local contraindication until it is completely healed. Clients who have had lymph nodes removed require special care due to the risk of lymphedema.

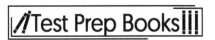
Special Populations
Some demographics require special consideration from healthcare providers. Massage is beneficial in most cases, but both the therapist and the client should be informed of any risks before treatment begins. Expectant mothers—especially during the first trimester of pregnancy—are a prime example of how complicated this issue can be.

Contraindications for Prenatal Massage
Massage therapy during the first trimester of pregnancy is a controversial issue. Other contraindications include the presence of pitting edema, which is usually a sign of **preeclampsia**. Preeclampsia is an extremely dangerous condition for which the expectant mother should seek immediate care from her physician.

In general, the therapist should also stay in communication with the client during treatment to be sure none of the techniques used are increasing common symptoms like nausea, headache, or swelling of the extremities. If a client reports an increase in any of these symptoms during a massage, the therapist should immediately switch to a different technique or end the session early.

Massage should never be performed on clients with high-risk pregnancies unless the clients have obtained medical clearance. It is important for therapists to conduct a thorough intake evaluation to assess each client's unique needs before beginning to work with a new prenatal client.

Tools
The majority of massage therapists enter the field fueled by their desire to help people. For this reason, it can be hard for therapists to turn clients away, even when they have some of the conditions listed in this guide. The following are some tools that can help a therapist work around a client's pre-existing health concerns:

Finger cots
These are small latex sheaths, meant to cover only one finger. They are especially useful if the therapist has a hangnail or a papercut and can still work but needs some extra protection. Full latex gloves are not only cumbersome, they also send a potentially upsetting message to the client. No one wants to receive massage from someone who perceives him or her as unclean. Finger cots are the best of both worlds.

Body pillows, towels, and bolsters
These are soft props that allow the therapist to position a client comfortably, even when he or she has an extremely limited range of motion. Body pillows are used for most prenatal massages, and towels and extra bolsters can be especially helpful for elderly clients or those with limited mobility.

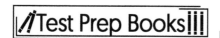

Special Applications

Special techniques can help clients with various chronic conditions. In some cases, the therapist will need an additional certification to perform these styles of bodywork. Here are some examples of massage styles that can relieve specific ailments:

- **Lymphatic Drainage:** a modality that focuses on circulating lymph throughout the body. The therapist uses an extremely light touch, stretching specific lymphatic vessels, thus stimulating flow. A special certification is recommended. This technique is contraindicated for hypertensive clients.

- **Craniosacral Therapy:** a light touch to manipulate the joints of the cranium, spine, and pelvis. This stimulates the natural flow of cerebrospinal fluid. This technique is similar to some styles of energy work.

- **Trigger Point Therapy (TRPT):** focused on very specific knots in any given muscle (aka, "trigger points"). TRPT allows the therapist to go in, release a painful adhesion, stretch the muscle, and move on. This is a popular method for relieving referred pain and headaches.

Areas of Caution

Areas of caution are specific anatomical areas of the body that require special consideration during bodywork. Some of these are unique to each client. As mentioned above, the therapist should never work directly over an open wound or any skin that is painful to the touch. Some clients have ticklish feet; some are uncomfortable with receiving work on their glutes (gluteus maximus). The therapist should clearly communicate with each client and be sure never to work on an area that will cause him or her more discomfort than benefit.

Additionally, the therapist should be cognizant of **endangerment sites,** areas that are sensitive on any human body, regardless of the client's personal preferences or conditions. The following areas contain major blood vessels, nerve bundles, and other structures that do not respond well to deep pressure during a massage:

- **Anterior Triangle of the Neck**—The area that contains major arteries and veins, including the jugular vein and the vagus nerve.

- **Posterior Triangle of the Neck**— The posterior triangle that offers access to the brachial plexus, which innervates most of the arm and hand. It contains major blood vessels.

- **Sternal Notch**—The area adjacent to the thyroid gland, which is responsible for regulating the endocrine system.

- **Axillary Area**—The armpit. It contains many major arteries as well as the brachial plexus.

- **Distal Humerus**—It contains the medial and lateral epicondyles of the humerus, which are adjacent to the ulnar and radial nerves, respectively, and has very little flesh to cushion pressure. It's sometimes called the "funny bone."

- **Abdomen**—It is home to most vital organs and the aorta, the largest blood vessel in the body, and requires therapists specially trained in abdominal massage.

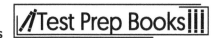
- **12th Rib**—The kidneys are almost entirely hidden by the 12th rib. Deep pressure (even to the tip of these organs) is extremely painful.

- **Sciatic Notch**—The sciatic nerve passes through the sciatic notch.

Areas of Caution

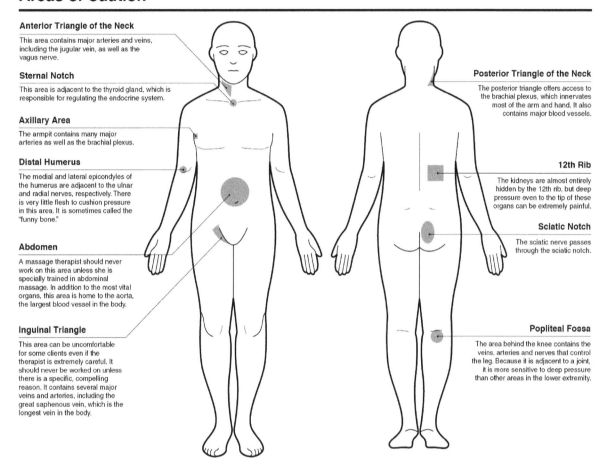

Anterior Triangle of the Neck
This area contains major arteries and veins, including the jugular vein, as well as the vagus nerve.

Sternal Notch
This area is adjacent to the thyroid gland, which is responsible for regulating the endocrine system.

Axillary Area
The armpit contains many major arteries as well as the brachial plexus.

Distal Humerus
The medial and lateral epicondyles of the humerus are adjacent to the ulnar and radial nerves, respectively. There is very little flesh to cushion pressure in this area. It is sometimes called the "funny bone."

Abdomen
A massage therapist should never work on this area unless she is specially trained in abdominal massage. In addition to the most vital organs, this area is home to the aorta, the largest blood vessel in the body.

Inguinal Triangle
This area can be uncomfortable for some clients even if the therapist is extremely careful. It should never be worked on unless there is a specific, compelling reason. It contains several major veins and arteries, including the great saphenous vein, which is the longest vein in the body.

Posterior Triangle of the Neck
The posterior triangle offers access to the brachial plexus, which innervates most of the arm and hand. It also contains major blood vessels.

12th Rib
The kidneys are almost entirely hidden by the 12th rib, but deep pressure even to the tip of these organs can be extremely painful.

Sciatic Notch
The sciatic nerve passes through the sciatic notch.

Popliteal Fossa
The area behind the knee contains the veins, arteries and nerves that control the leg. Because it is adjacent to a joint, it is more sensitive to deep pressure than other areas in the lower extremity.

- **Inguinal Triangle**—It contains several major veins and arteries, including the great saphenous vein, which is the longest vein in the body. It is uncomfortable for some clients, even if the therapist is extremely careful. It should never be worked on without a specific, compelling reason.

- **Popliteal Fossa**—The area behind the knee that contains the veins, arteries, and nerves that control the leg. It is adjacent to a joint, making it more sensitive to deep pressure than other areas in the lower extremity.

Special Populations

As mentioned, some demographics require special consideration from healthcare providers. Massage is beneficial in most cases, but both the therapist and the client should be informed of any risks before treatment begins.

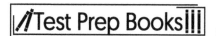

Prenatal Massage

Prenatal massage requires the therapist to be well-versed in the physical changes that come with the different stages of pregnancy. Each trimester comes with its own unique challenges, and it is important for any massage therapist to anticipate the needs of the client—especially for women who are pregnant for the first time and may not know what is "normal."

The first trimester of any pregnancy carries a high risk of miscarriage, and for that reason, many massage therapists choose not to perform massage on newly pregnant women until that dangerous time has passed. The question of whether massage can cause miscarriage is a controversial one. Although recent studies seem to suggest that massage does *not* increase the risk of miscarriage, this commonly held belief may make a therapist legally vulnerable should anything go awry.

Past a certain point, it will be uncomfortable for the client to lie supine or prone. From then on, the therapist should plan to perform massage on the client in a side-lying position, which requires special draping techniques and body pillows. The therapist should also learn about pressure points associated with inducing labor and avoid them while performing prenatal work. Note that these pressure points can only be accessed from very specific angles and that effleurage over the general area is usually safe. The following techniques can be particularly helpful:

- Palpation of pressure points to relieve nausea (for clients experiencing morning sickness)
- Lymphatic drainage (for clients with edema)
- Tractioning of the lumbar spine

Although it is legal for any licensed massage therapist to perform this kind of work, certification in prenatal massage is highly recommended.

Infants

Massage can be just as beneficial for infants as it is for adults, albeit for different reasons. Infants have a highly developed sense of touch. They need to be touched often so that they learn how to bond with other people. When working on an infant, it is best to invite the parent into the room throughout the session. This calms the baby down and also aids in communication. Because the infant cannot speak in words to explain how he/she feels or if something hurts, the therapist must rely on body language, facial expression, and the intuition of the people who know the infant best.

Massage for infants should be extremely gentle, and sessions should be shorter than they are for adults; no longer than twenty minutes is recommended.

Elderly Clients

The elderly population faces a unique kind of discrimination in some Western cultures. People living in nursing homes and hospice care rarely experience touch, especially the compassionate, nurturing touch offered by a massage therapist. Massage can reduce the stress and anxiety of daily life, improve digestive function, and stimulate blood flow and muscle growth for even the most sedentary clients. This is especially helpful when working with clients who live with chronic conditions that prevent them from engaging in strenuous physical exercise. Simply connecting with any client as a friendly healthcare provider can give him or her something to look forward to; for the elderly, that spark of hope and excitement can make a huge difference in their overall health.

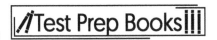
When working with these clients, it is especially important to approach them with respect and flexibility. Massage therapists who have worked in nursing homes report the importance of patience with clients who have limited mobility and take a longer time to undress. Some people may need the therapist to travel to the home or a hospital room. For clients with hearing or sight impairments, the massage therapist may need to find creative ways of announcing their presence.

Perhaps most important is that the massage therapist pay attention to each client's cognitive function. Many elders are treated poorly because younger people assume that they have lost their intellect along with their mobility. This is not only rude, it is discriminatory. However, for clients who do suffer from Alzheimer's or other forms of dementia, the therapist should be ready to meet them anew in every session in a patient, calm, and kind manner.

Disabled Clients

Disabilities come in many forms. Massage therapy can be helpful for people with a wide variety of chronic ailments, including developmental disabilities; neurological dysfunctions, such as cerebral palsy; and physical limitations like paralysis.

Each of these populations requires a unique understanding from any healthcare provider. Working with clients who have developmental disabilities often means the therapist must travel to them and learn to communicate with great patience. People who do not speak or make eye contact might not respond well to a forceful "Hello!" and the offer of a handshake. The therapist must meet these clients halfway and learn to communicate with them in a way that they can understand.

Many disabled people experience touch in a different way than others do. Severely autistic people, for example, can find gentle touch overwhelming and upsetting but usually respond well to very deep pressure. It is important to spend time getting to know each client and learning how to meet their specific needs.

For clients with physical disabilities, especially clients who are wheelchair bound, massage can greatly improve quality of life. Lymphatic techniques and effleurage stimulate blood flow, even to and from limbs that cannot move. Myofascial release can reduce any tension or pain due to large areas of scar tissue. Massage may not be able to treat the initial condition that causes immobility or pain (such as an injury to the spinal cord), but it can go a long way toward relieving a client's ongoing symptoms.

Oncology Clients

Clients with cancer require a very special type of care. The therapist who deals with this population should most certainly be educated and certified in oncology massage. While there is a great deal of medical and technical knowledge that one must have to safely massage a client with cancer, it is also important to show an extra level of compassion and care, as they are dealing with very stressful situations and, in many cases, may be fighting for their lives.

Classes of Medications

Pharmacology
Pharmacology is the study of drugs and their physiological effects. Ongoing research looks at the effectiveness of various substances for treating a particular disease, while causing the fewest and least harmful side effects. Massage therapists must be familiar with commonly used drugs and remain well-informed as medical protocols change.

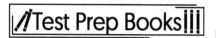

Definition of Drug

A **drug** is defined as any chemical that is ingested or enters the body in some form and results in a physiological change in the body. There are countless examples of drugs in our society. Legal drugs are prescribed to treat cancer, hypertension, pain, digestive disorders, and so on. Illegal drugs are also in use; even caffeine is a drug.

Classifying Drugs

Drugs come in many forms. Many different drugs with similar physiological effects have vastly different names, uses, and side effects. For example, a person experiencing pain may first seek an over-the-counter drug like Advil because it is inexpensive, readily available, and has few adverse side effects with short-term use. If he or she needs a less expensive version of the same drug, the generic ibuprofen may be an option. The drug in both cases is ibuprofen; Advil is just a brand name. The only difference between the two drugs is their packaging. If over-the-counter drugs are not strong enough to treat the person's pain, he or she should consult a doctor. It is likely that the doctor will prescribe opiates to treat the pain in the short term, with a long-term plan to address the underlying cause of discomfort. **Opiates** are much stronger than over-the-counter drugs. They are also highly addictive, and long-term use can result in serious physical and mental health problems. Like ibuprofen, opiates come with many names. For example, hydrocodone may be packaged as Vicodin or Norco. This is just one example of the myriad of ways that drugs are named, classified, and distributed.

Massage therapists should familiarize themselves with drugs commonly used to treat pain, muscle spasms, and other common maladies such as hypertension and hypocholesteremia. Armed with as much knowledge as possible, the therapist can make an informed decision about whether massage is safe for the client.

Anti-Anxiety Drugs

Anti-anxiety drugs are prescribed to people who experience occasional panic attacks or a persistent and chronic state of anxiety. Many antidepressants (listed below) are also used to alleviate anxiety. If a client is taking a drug specifically for anxiety and one *not* intended to treat depression, it will likely be a benzodiazepine.

Benzodiazepines: drugs intended to decrease stress and feelings of anxiety. These drugs can also function as muscle relaxants. In high doses, they can induce sleep or non-responsiveness; massage therapists should proceed with caution when working on clients who regularly take benzodiazepines. Some examples include Diazepam (branded as Valium), Lorazepam (branded as Ativan), and Alprazolam (branded as Xanax).

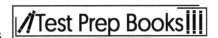
Antidepressants

Antidepressants are designed to increase energy levels, alleviate sluggishness and despondency, and help people with depression live happier, healthier lives. Common side effects of antidepressants include nausea, loss of sex drive, and weight gain. The different classes of antidepressants impact the brain in various ways:

- **Selective Serotonin Reuptake Inhibitors (SSRIs):** By far the most commonly prescribed class of antidepressant, SSRIs make extracellular serotonin more readily available, increasing and regulating its effect on the brain. Some examples are Prozac, Celexa, and Lexapro.

- **Selective Norepinephrine Reuptake Inhibitors (SNRIs):** Similar to SSRIs in most ways, these drugs also prevent the re-uptake of **norepinephrine**, a chemical related to adrenaline. Some examples are Effexor and Cymbalta.

- **Tricyclic Antidepressants:** These are some of the oldest antidepressants on the market and come with many more side effects than SSRIs. They prevent the re-uptake of serotonin, norepinephrine, and some dopamine. Some examples are Anafranil and Norpramin.

- **Atypical Antidepressants:** These drugs have various mechanisms for treating depression. Some examples are Wellbutrin, Remeron, and Serzone.

Anti-Inflammatories and Analgesics

Analgesics, or painkillers, reduce pain but do not treat the root cause. Some analgesics work by reducing inflammation while others act directly on the nervous system. Massage is contraindicated for clients actively taking analgesics because these drugs make it impossible to know when the therapist's pressure is excessive. There are four main classes of analgesics:

- **Non-narcotic Analgesics:** These drugs are often available over the counter. An example is acetaminophen (found in Tylenol and DayQuil).

- **Non-Steroidal Anti-Inflammatory Drugs (NSAIDs):** These are over-the-counter drugs that reduce inflammation, therefore reducing pain. Long-term use can damage the lining of the stomach, causing ulcers. Some examples are aspirin (found in Acuprin and Bufferin) and ibuprofen (found in Advil and Motrin).

- **COX-2 Inhibitors:** Derived from NSAIDs, these drugs only inhibit COX-2 enzymes (whereas NSAIDs inhibit both COX-1 and COX-2). They have similar effects, but are not as harmful to the stomach lining. An example is celecoxib (found in Celebrex).

- **Opioids (narcotic analgesics):** These prescription drugs are derived from opium and are highly addictive. Long-term use can cause physical and emotional problems. They impact the nervous system by blocking **nociceptors** (pain receptors) in the brain from recognizing pain signals. Some examples include hydrocodone (found in Vicodin) and oxycodone (found in OxyContin and Roxicodone).

Autonomic Nervous System Disorder Medications

The **autonomic nervous system (ANS)** is the division of the nervous system responsible for involuntary functions, including the fight-or-flight response governed by the sympathetic nervous system and the

63

rest-and-digest reactions of the parasympathetic nervous system. Massage is known to stimulate the parasympathetic nervous system. This process promotes good digestion, deep breathing, more effective oxygenation of the blood, relaxation of the muscles, and the release of neurotransmitters responsible for happiness and pleasure. A client with an ongoing disorder of the ANS might have an atypical response to massage. The following drugs may be listed on an intake form for such a client:

- **Cholinergic drugs:** These drugs are also called **parasympathomimetic drugs** because they mimic the normal activity of the neurotransmitter acetylcholine in a healthy parasympathetic nervous system. These drugs are prescribed to people with disorders such as myasthenia gravis, glaucoma, and bladder dysfunction. Some examples include Urecholine, Arecholine, and Carbachol.

- **Anticholinergic drugs:** These drugs block acetylcholine receptors in the ANS, relieving involuntary muscle spasms, among other symptoms. They are often prescribed for people suffering from GI disorders, asthma, and some symptoms of Parkinson's disease. Some examples are clozapine, Seroquel, and some antipsychotics.

- **Adrenergic drugs:** Sometimes referred to as **sympathomimetic drugs**, these drugs bolster the sympathetic nervous system's activity. They regulate neurotransmitters released in fight-or-flight situations, such as adrenaline and noradrenaline. They are used to increase blood flow and oxygen exchange, usually during medical crises like allergic reactions or asthma attacks. Some examples are Albuterol, Epinephrine, and Ephedrine.

- **Antiadrenergic drugs:** Also called **sympatholytic drugs**, these drugs inhibit some functions of the sympathetic nervous system. They are used to treat various disorders, including anxiety and hypertension. Some examples include Acebutolol, Doxazosin, and Clonidine.

Cardiovascular Drugs

There are many different drugs for cardiovascular disease. These are prescribed to people who have (or are at risk for) heart attacks and hypertension:

- **Angiotensin-Converting Enzyme (ACE) Inhibitors:** These drugs lower angiotensin II levels, effectively decreasing resistance in blood vessels. Some examples are Benazepril, Captopril, and Enalapril.

- **Angiotensin II Receptor Blockers (ARBs):** ARBs have a similar effect to ACE inhibitors, using a different mechanism. They prevent the body from absorbing angiotensin II. Some examples are Candesartan, Losartan, and Valsartan.

- **Beta Blockers:** These drugs decrease heart rate, thus reducing the volume of blood pumping through arteries at any given time and lowering blood pressure. Examples include Acebutolol, Atenolol, Propranolol, and Nadolol.

- **Calcium Blockers:** By interrupting the flow of calcium through the blood vessels, these drugs help the heart pump less forcefully, which can reduce workload on the heart. Some examples are Felodipine, Verapamil, and Nifedipine.

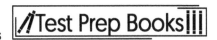

- **Digitoxin:** These drugs, such as Lanoxin, help the heart pump more powerfully. This can be useful for patients who have congestive heart failure.

- **Diuretics:** These drugs increase the volume of urine, thus decreasing excess fluids from the body and relieving strain on the cardiovascular system. Some examples are Amiloride, Bumetanide, and Indapamide.

Cancer Drugs

Chemotherapy refers to the treatment of disease using chemical agents. In the United States, the term is used specifically to describe drugs that attack cancerous cells. Unfortunately, chemotherapy drugs do not yet solely target cancerous cells. They attack all cells in the body with the intent of killing cancer cells before destroying healthy cells. A client undergoing chemotherapy may experience many severe and dangerous side effects.

- **Alkylating agents:** These powerful drugs attack the DNA of cancerous cells, killing them and preventing them from reproducing. Some examples are mechlorethamine, chlorambucil, streptozocin, and Temodar.

- **Antimetabolites:** These drugs are commonly used to treat leukemia and breast cancer, as they interrupt the reproductive process of cancerous cells. Some examples are 5-FU, Xeloda, Hydroxyurea, and Alimta.

- **Anti-tumor Antibiotics:** Unlike the antibiotics used to treat bacterial infections, these drugs interrupt the functioning of DNA at all stages of the cell cycle. Some examples are Adriamycin, Epirubicin, Idarubicin, and Bleomycin.

- **Topoisomerase Inhibitors:** These drugs target the enzymes that help organize strands of DNA. Some examples are Topotecan and Etoposide.

- **Mitotic Inhibitors:** These drugs prevent enzymes from making proteins to build more cells, thus interrupting cell reproduction. Some examples are Ixempra, Velban, and Emcyt.

Clot Management Drugs

People with hypertension, clotting disorders (like DVT), or congenital heart defects may be prescribed blood thinners. These drugs manage the body's ability to form blood clots. A common side effect is excessive bleeding because the patient will have difficulty forming scabs over any wound. The two most common classes of blood thinners are anticoagulants and antiplatelet drugs:

- **Anticoagulants:** These drugs slow the clotting (**coagulation**) process. Some examples are heparin and Coumadin (aka Warfarin).

- **Antiplatelet drugs:** These drugs prevent platelets (one kind of blood cell) from sticking together and forming clots. An example is aspirin.

Diabetes Management Drugs

Diabetes is a condition in which the body is unable to properly regulate glucose levels in the blood. This can either be due to a lack of insulin produced by the pancreas (**Type I**) or, more commonly in the United States, from an inability of the cells to effectively use insulin (**Type II**), known as insulin-resistance. Type II Diabetes is, unfortunately, very common in the American adult population due to the increase in obesity and unhealthy lifestyles. Diabetic clients may have a very specific diet and exercise regime and are often prescribed drugs to manage the disease.

Most commonly, diabetics are prescribed one of the following:

IV pumps help diabetics control their insulin levels on the go

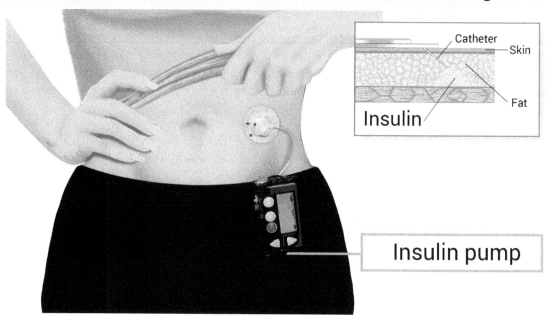

- **Insulin:** This is a hormone naturally produced in the pancreas that diabetic clients either lack or cannot effectively regulate and respond to. Insulin is administered intravenously, and clients may have regular injections or a constant drip via an insulin pump. Therapists should not work directly over the site of injection.

- **Oral glucose management drugs:** These drugs come in many forms and are most often prescribed to people with Type II Diabetes. They also serve to regulate insulin, often by inhibiting its production in the pancreas. Some examples are Amaryl, Diabeta, and Metformin.

Muscle Relaxants

Muscle relaxants are used to temporarily relieve pain and tension in skeletal muscles. Like most analgesics, these drugs do not treat the cause of the pain: they merely alleviate the symptoms. Muscle relaxants work in one of two ways:

- **Centrally-acting muscle relaxants:** These drugs slow brain activity and inhibit **nociception**—the process through which the brain perceives pain. Side effects can include drowsiness, sluggishness, and nausea. Some examples are Valium, Flexeril, and Soma.

- **Peripherally-acting muscle relaxants:** These drugs, such as Dantrium, act directly on the spasming muscle or muscles and can cause temporary instability.

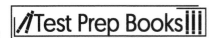
Thyroid Supplement Drugs

Drugs and supplements can be prescribed to treat clients with hyperthyroidism or hypothyroidism. **Hyperthyroidism** is most often treated with beta blockers (described above, under cardiovascular drugs) or surgery. **Hypothyroidism**—when the thyroid is underactive—can be treated with a number of drugs including:

- **Levothyroxine:** A synthetic compound that provides the body with more of the hormones T3 and T4, which are naturally produced by a healthy thyroid. Some examples are Synthroid, Levoxyl, and Unithroid.

- **Desiccated Thyroid Extract:** A natural version of levothyroxine that has similar effects. Desiccated Thyroid Extract is made from the thyroid glands of pigs or cows. Some examples are Naturethroid and Westhroid.

Herbal Supplements and Vitamins

Herbs and supplements are natural drugs made from plants, vitamins, and minerals. Most are available over-the-counter, which means that clients may take them without the supervision of a healthcare professional. Examples include vitamin C, iron supplements, folic acid, fish oil, magnesium, and probiotics.

Herbs can also be prescribed by acupuncturists and other healthcare providers for very specific purposes. These natural remedies have been in use for thousands of years and long before the pharmaceutical industry existed. They can be extremely potent and can interact in various ways with other drugs the client is taking.

Benefits and Effects of Techniques that Manipulate Soft Tissue

Identification of the Physiological Effects of Soft Tissue Manipulation

Massage serves many purposes, including relaxation and more pointed, specific work. Even for therapists who only offer relaxation massages, a detailed understanding of anatomy and physiology is essential. Anatomy is the study of the location and physical structure of body structures. For instance, the rotator cuff muscles (supraspinatus, infraspinatus, teres minor, and subscapularis) all attach to and help stabilize the shoulder. **Physiology** is the study of how the structures and systems of the body work, such as the exchange of oxygen that occurs in the alveoli of the lungs. Because of the intimate relationship between the two, massage therapists must have a good understanding of both sciences to be optimal clinicians. For example, to fully understand why friction techniques help ease scar tissue, one must understand both the anatomy of scar tissue and healthy muscle as well as the physiology of the inflammatory and healing process. This is true for even the simplest techniques.

Effects on Muscular Structure
Of all the body's systems, the skeletal system is the one that is most directly impacted by massage. Massage increases blood flow, which brings more oxygen and nutrients to areas of pain. It also draws the client's attention to old injuries, encouraging them to release tension they may be holding subconsciously. Deeper techniques, such as friction, can break up scar tissue and reorganize muscle fibers and adhesions so that fibers are properly aligned for optimal function.

Effects on the Nervous System
Many massage techniques are designed specifically to invoke a particular stimulus to the nervous system. **Trigger point therapy**, for instance, reminds the brain of old injuries, increasing the activity of the nociceptors at the site. The brain responds to this afferent sensory input and increases blood flow to the area to help heal the tissue. One deep friction technique called "**clearing**" gradually increases pain in the area until the Golgi tendon organs become overwhelmed and shut down. Although it is initially painful, this process deeply relaxes even the most hypertonic muscles. Percussive strokes can "wake up" the nervous system and increase a client's energy, while long gentle strokes can relax neural signaling and soothe a client to sleep.

Effects on the Autonomic Nervous System
Beyond its impact on specific areas, massage stimulates the autonomic nervous system in truly remarkable ways. The ANS is divided into two branches: the **sympathetic nervous system**, which controls the fight-or-flight response, and the **parasympathetic nervous system** (or PSNS), which is responsible for rest-and-digest functions. Massage specifically stimulates the PSNS, promoting healthy digestion, encouraging deeper and more effective breathing, and decreasing stress.

Effects on the Circulatory System
Massage increases the flow of all fluids in the body. Blood flow is increased, which brings more oxygen and nutrients to the muscles and organs. The flow of lymph is also stimulated, helping the body process and eliminate waste more effectively. Lymphatic drainage is a specific form of massage designed to

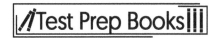
relieve pain by increasing lymphatic flow without directly impacting skeletal muscles. The influx of fluids to the circulatory system is beneficial for most clients but can be dangerous for those with hypertension.

Pain Relief
Physical pain comes in many forms. **Acute muscle pain** is typically caused by injury. Examples of acute pain are whiplash from a car accident or a "pulled" muscle from a slip on the soccer field. Acute injuries can even be caused by actions that don't feel painful at the time, such as the gradual onset of muscle soreness induced by unaccustomed activity, such as moving apartments. Massage can greatly relieve symptoms caused by injuries like these.

Psychological Aspects and Benefits of Touch

Touch, or skin-to-skin contact between any two people, is an essential part of massage therapy. Simply touching someone releases serotonin, oxytocin, and dopamine in both people, promoting a sense of happiness and safety. Furthermore, touch is essential in any human being's process of forming attachments. The more humans touch and are touched by other people, the easier it is to treat themselves, their families, and their loved ones with compassion and respect. This simple action is a powerful tool for healing and for life in general.

Pain Management
Chronic pain is far more insidious and challenging to heal than acute pain. For example, a mother who carries her 20-pound toddler on a daily basis, a person who works at a desk ill-suited to their body, or a dentist who spends the work day contorted over a patient's body all might have chronic muscle injuries sustained in the course of their daily activities. Massage is helpful in easing both acute and chronic pain, although different techniques should be used in each case. Massage can also improve a client's general body awareness. Encouraging proper body mechanics can greatly diminish chronic pain.

Stress
Constant physical or emotional stress can damage a muscle. Clearly, the stress of a physically demanding job builds up over time and causes pain. Emotional stress can have the same effect. Increased levels of cortisol, epinephrine, and norepinephrine make muscles tight and painful. A lack of restful sleep decreases the body's ability to heal itself. By releasing dopamine, serotonin, and oxytocin, massage can improve the balance of neurotransmitters in the body. Although a massage therapist cannot directly remove external stressors, bodywork can inspire hope and a sense of well-being.

Differentiation Between Pain and Stress
Pain is a perceived sensation that gets transmitted to the Central Nervous System (CNS) by nociceptors. If the body is considered to be a well-oiled machine, pain can be envisioned as an alarm going off when a part is damaged. Pain alerts the individual to stop the painful activity. Chronic pain and stress have similar effects on the body. Stress is defined as tension or strain that can be either physical or emotional in nature. Most stress stems from long-term issues, such as high-pressure work environments, family or financial instability, or even chronic pain. Clearly, stress and pain are closely linked and one can influence the other. A massage therapist cannot remove the stressors from clients' lives as it is outside the scope of practice of LMTs to help clients quit their jobs or leave abusive relationships. However, the relief from physical pain induced by a good massage can go a long way toward relieving even the most severe forms of stress.

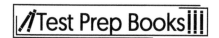

Distinguishing Between Acute and Chronic Pain

Acute and chronic pain are designated as such based on the timeline of an injury. **Acute pain** comes on quickly – one moment the client is pain-free, then the next moment they are hurting. A car accident, a fall, or a nap on an uncomfortable couch can all result in acute pain. **Chronic pain** is defined as pain that lasts for more than 6 weeks. Chronic pain can result from an acute injury that heals improperly or from misuse of a muscle over a long time. People who work at desks often have chronic neck pain due to anterior head carriage; many expectant mothers have chronic low back pain caused by abdominal weight gain. If a client seeks medical attention as soon as they notice acute pain, the healing process is often linear, and they can usually expect a full recovery. Clients seeking treatment for chronic pain have a more complicated healing trajectory. Their recovery is not always linear, and they must implement major changes in their body mechanics in order to correct the ongoing issue.

Dopamine, Serotonin, and Oxytocin

Skin-to-skin contact of any kind stimulates the production of dopamine, serotonin, and oxytocin. Massage has been clinically proven to have a significant positive effect on these three neurotransmitters.

- **Serotonin** increases feelings of happiness and well-being. It also aids in the regulation of appetite and healthy sleep patterns. It is stimulated by things such as physical touch, professional success, happy memories, and sunlight.

- **Dopamine** is responsible for pleasure and motivation. Its production is increased by any kind of physical touch, consuming alcohol or any addictive substance, and completing important tasks.

- **Oxytocin**, often called "the love hormone," is instrumental in the ability of humans to bond with each other. It is primarily stimulated by touch and can reach extremely high levels in nursing mothers, helping the baby bond with the mother.

These neurotransmitters are essential for positive mental health, happiness, and overall well-being. Any physical touch can increase dopamine, serotonin, and oxytocin levels, but massage is particularly effective.

Benefits of Soft Tissue Manipulation for Specific Client Populations

Massage is helpful for people from all walks of life. Certain groups can benefit from bodywork in unique ways. Here are just a few examples of specific client populations that may find massage especially important in their healing process.

Trauma Survivors

Survivors of any trauma, from sexual assault to severe car accidents, must often work hard to reconnect with their bodies. Massage can be a gentle way to begin and assist this process. Massage improves body awareness naturally, and conversations with a massage therapist can help survivors learn how to think about their healing process. For people healing from physical trauma like surgical procedures, massage is an opportunity to get needed professional care without experiencing even more pain. It's common for clients to dread sessions with a physical therapist, but it's quite rare for a returning client to dread their massage. Regular sessions can help patients mark the timeline of their healing process. It is very encouraging for a client to hear their therapist remark, "Wow, your range of motion is vastly improved since last week!" Unfortunately, healing is not linear. Even when clients experience setbacks, discussing

70

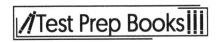

their process with a massage therapist can help them feel supported. This kind of teamwork and emotional validation is vital for any kind of healing.

Recovering Clients Who Struggle with Addiction

Clients who seek treatment for addiction have likely been through a crisis. Relatively few people choose to quit drinking or using drugs just because they feel like it. Consequently, these individuals are not only healing physically (and possibly experiencing withdrawal symptoms), but they are also probably rebuilding their lives and relationships from the ground up. A massage therapist, or any healthcare provider, can offer a great deal of solace. Just by being present, listening to them, and keeping reliable boundaries, a provider can help these clients re-learn how to form healthy relationships. Physically, individuals who struggle with addiction are accustomed to getting a rush of dopamine whenever they use their drug of choice. As described, **dopamine** is a naturally-occurring neurotransmitter necessary for feelings of happiness. Any person recovering from addiction must learn how to increase levels of this important chemical from healthier sources. Massage is one such source. Working with a massage therapist can have a neurochemical impact on any person's ability to be happy. This is especially true for those in recovery.

Elderly Clients

Unfortunately, Western culture tends to treat elderly people as invisible. They are banished from the workplace and isolated in nursing homes, and they are viewed as untouchable. Subsequently, it is very difficult to go from a life filled with friendly hugs, romantic embraces, and even professional handshakes, to the isolation of a nursing home. For this reason, massage can be extremely helpful in the physical and mental health of the elderly population. Massage therapists are trained to treat every client with the utmost respect, regardless of their age, physical appearance, or body odor. All bodies deserve professional attention. Massage therapists can offer elderly clients an opportunity to reconnect with their bodies, as they relieve the aches and pains of daily life and stimulate the positive feelings associated with physical touch.

New Mothers

Prenatal massage is a booming industry, but there are also many benefits of post-natal massage. New mothers, especially first-time mothers, experience major physical changes. While their bodies must recover from the stress of pregnancy and delivery, they simultaneously begin to care for a newborn. Their sleep patterns are unpredictable and rarely restful. Their posture changes to accommodate nursing, and they experience upper body fatigue due to carrying the baby, diapers, toys, bottles, and so forth. This process essentially happens overnight and it can be physically painful. Massage can serve many purposes in the life of a new mother. It can help relieve the pain of muscle growth and weight loss or gain, improve body awareness and help the client improve posture, and even be a valuable opportunity for the new mother to take a nap. A regular routine of bodywork also offers some consistency in her hectic life; this can be extremely important for positive mental health.

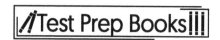

Soft Tissue Techniques

Types of Strokes

Massage strokes vary between styles of bodywork. Clinical work, for instance, will involve far more traction; relaxation massage might use more aromatherapy. However, there are some basic movements that translate across all techniques:

- **Touch:** static contact between the therapist and the client. Minimal pressure is necessary.

- **Stroking:** gently moving the hands across a broad area of skin, such as the entire back. No pressure is applied; the therapist should use a light, feathery touch.

- **Effleurage:** a gliding stroke with constant pressure. The therapist should apply a firm touch, without reaching any depth within the muscle. This word is derived from the French term "to glide."

- **Petrissage:** derived from the French "to knead." Petrissage is specific, deep-tissue work, focused on a particular muscle or knot.

- **Tapotement:** percussive techniques (from the French "to strike"). These strokes should be quick and well-aimed. The client should feel invigorated but never bruised.

- **Joint mobilizations:** the movement of a joint, by the therapist, through its pain-free range of motion. This technique gently relaxes several muscle groups simultaneously and draws the client's awareness to the limb.

Sequence of Application

During a massage session, timing is of the utmost importance. A therapist working in a spa uses different techniques than someone working in a hospital or a chiropractor's office. Similarly, treating a client for acute muscle spasms requires different strategies than treating the same client for emotional stress. The therapist should always be mindful of the clock and should be sure to spend the proper amount of time working on each area of the body. Here are some general rules to follow that will help with the timing and flow of a massage:

Resting Position

Every massage should begin with stillness. The therapist should place their hands on the client's body and ask them to breathe deeply, and both individuals should work on relaxing. This posture should be maintained until both parties are ready to begin the massage. It may take 5 seconds or 5 minutes. The therapist should experiment with pressure, timing, and personal emotional intentions during resting positions.

General/Specific/General

This protocol will guide you throughout a massage session and throughout a long-term relationship with a client. Many of the protocols listed below are simply more detailed versions of this basic idea. Therapists can implement this idea by first working generally, such as applying compressions to the client's entire body or stroking the entire back. Myofascial release across a broad area, such as the back or an entire limb, is a good way to do general work. Next, specific work is addressed. Using the example of the back, after stroking, effleurage may begin in the upper left quadrant, warming the trapezius, the

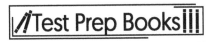
erector spinae, and latissimus dorsi. The work becomes increasingly specific, leading into trigger point therapy or other forms of petrissage to release the root cause of the client's pain.

Once all of the intended specific work is completed, the LMT should slowly work back toward more general techniques and finish the session with stroking, compressions, or traction techniques. This process is slow and gentle. It is important to follow this protocol because it protects the muscles against shock. The client gets used to the therapist's pressure over a long period of time, and, as a result, they are able to withstand much deeper and more specific work.

Superficial/Deep/Superficial

Another aspect of the general/specific/general idea, this protocol refers to the therapist's pressure. Massages should never begin with trigger point therapy. Instead, stroking or effleurage will help warm the muscles and release the connective tissue. Once the surrounding area is warm enough to relax around the site of pain, the therapist can go in more deeply and effectively, focusing on a specific injury without causing unnecessary pain.

Proximal/Distal/Proximal

This protocol refers to work on a limb. Because blood flows from the heart outward to the extremities, it is important to open up proximal areas of a limb before working distally. That way, the muscles around veins and arteries are released and blood can circulate throughout the distal area of pain, instead of pooling around a joint. For example, if a client has shin splints, the therapist should begin work at the hip flexors, releasing all muscle tissue in the quadriceps and around the knee before arriving at the site of pain.

Peripheral/Central/Peripheral

This protocol is similar to the proximal/distal/proximal strategy, but applied to the torso or any specific injury in a broad muscle. For example, if a client has trigger points in the trapezius that cause headaches, the LMT should start by working on the entire muscle, from the occiput to the shoulders and then down to the thoracic attachment. The therapist should work on releasing any myofascial adhesions and use long effleurage strokes to lengthen the muscle in all three fiber directions. Once the muscle has begun to relax, specific trigger points causing referred pain can be addressed. At this point, the surrounding tissue should have enough elasticity that the knots can relax back into their ideal alignment. Finally, the therapist should go back over the entire muscle, smoothing any tightness that formed during trigger point therapy.

Stretching

This is an important part of any treatment, even when relaxation is the only goal. Stretching specific muscles after deep effleurage and petrissage reminds the brain of proper alignment and encourages muscle fibers to relax into that position. This is especially important after abrasive work, such as a friction massage, but it is helpful in any situation.

Breathing

Throughout a massage, the therapist should be aware of the client's breathing patterns as well as their own. Deep breathing improves oxygen exchange in the lungs, which means blood can bring oxygen and other nutrients to the muscles more efficiently. This is important self-care for the therapist and client alike. Also, when a therapist breathes deeply, it naturally inspires the client to do the same. Finally, a therapist can listen to the client's breathing for important clues about pressure. For instance, if a client

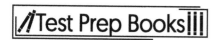

suddenly catches their breath or sucks in air through their teeth, it is often a sign that the pressure has gone too deep too fast, and the therapist should adjust accordingly.

Overview of Massage/Bodywork Modalities

There are many modalities that one can master as a massage therapist. The more knowledgeable and well-rounded a therapist is, the more effective their work will be. This section will explore several common modalities, but it is not a comprehensive list.

Swedish Massage

This is the most popular style of massage, especially at spas. It is a relaxing modality that uses medium pressure and continuous flowing movements. The techniques used during Swedish massage include effleurage, petrissage, tapotement, and friction.

Deep Tissue Massage

This modality uses an overall deeper pressure but focuses on specific muscle groups and trigger points. Slow, deep strokes and stretching techniques release tension from the deeper layers of muscle tissue. It is important to communicate with clients throughout this type of massage to determine their comfort level and whether the pressure is too forceful or deep. This modality has a number of contraindications, including certain recent injuries, unregulated high blood pressure, and diabetes, so it is important for the therapist to gather a thorough health history prior to administering this technique.

Sports Massage

This type of massage is intended for athletes. Different styles of sports massage are offered before, during, and after an athletic competition. Every sports massage is unique and should be tailored to the athlete's specific needs. The sports massage therapist should be trained in treating as many injuries as possible, since it is impossible to know what will arise during a sporting event. Contrary to popular belief, sports massage does not always involve deep tissue work. Instead, it uses many different techniques to reduce muscle fatigue and pain, stimulate blood flow and circulation, and improve flexibility and posture.

Along with basic techniques such as effleurage, tapotement, and petrissage, sports massage uses cross friction, compressions, passive and active stretching, range of motion work, and vibration. As with any modality, communication with the client before, during, and after a sports massage is imperative. The therapist must be familiar with the basics of each sport to determine which muscle groups are most affected for a given athlete. Checking in with the athlete during the massage helps the therapist know if he or she is helping the client or causing unnecessary pain.

Here's a sports massage being performed:

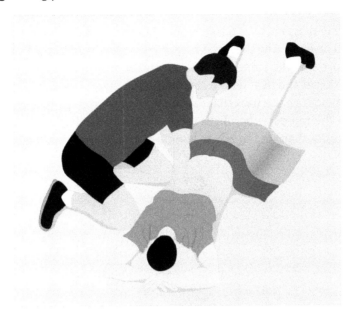

Chair Massage

The primary benefit of **chair massage** is its mobility. It is often conducted in airports, malls, sporting events, and even corporate offices. These massages are typically 10-20 minutes, which enables therapists to address some of a client's issues without going into great detail. Chair massage is most often used as a promotional tool for either a particular massage therapist or a business that offers massage therapy. The client remains fully clothed as the therapist works the upper posterior body, the neck, and/or the arms. Proper body mechanics are extremely important for the massage therapist during chair massage.

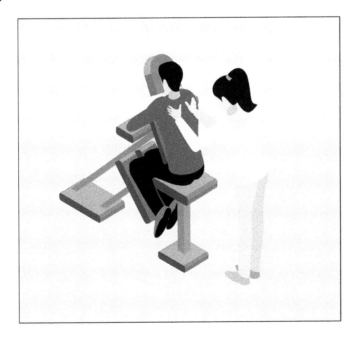

75

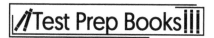
Hot Stone Massage

Modern Western hot stone massage uses basalt stones heated in a stone warmer or crock pot filled with water heated to 120-150 degrees. The therapist begins with some traditional Swedish massage to lubricate the skin to ensure that the stones glide comfortably over the muscles. **Hot stone massage** is slow, rhythmic, and relaxing as the heat penetrates to deeper layers of muscle. The therapist might place stones on various points on the back, hands, and feet to encourage relaxation. It is vital to check in with the client regarding the temperature of the stones to avoid skin burns. A bowl of cold water is also recommended to cool stones that are too hot to handle or to use safely on the body.

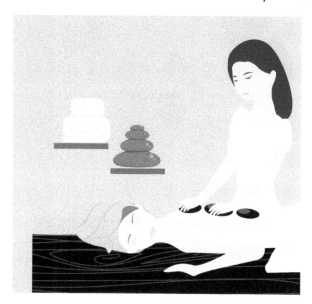

Thai Massage

Thai massage or **Thai yoga massage** consists of a series of passive stretching and compression techniques that work the entire body, including all muscles, tendons, and organ systems. This particular modality is good for stress reduction, increased flexibility, blood flow, range of motion, and relaxation. Rooted in Ayurvedic traditions, the belief is that it works along the body's energy pathways to clear blockages and restore balance. Considered more bodywork than massage, Thai yoga massage uses a series of assisted yoga positions on a floor mat, with the client fully clothed in loose, comfortable attire.

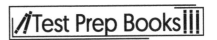
Prenatal/Pregnancy Massage

Prenatal massage has been shown to help with many of the physical and emotional stressors encountered during pregnancy. First and foremost, massage helps to relax busy expecting mothers. This lowers cortisol levels, which directly correlates with improved health for the baby.

Prenatal massage can also relieve pain caused by pregnancy-induced edema and sciatica. Edema, or fluid retention and swelling in the extremities, is another pregnancy symptom targeted by prenatal massage, which can help by improving circulation and fluid drainage in swollen tissues and joints. Sciatica can be caused when the extra weight from the baby puts pressure on the sciatic nerve, causing very uncomfortable and sometimes debilitating pain. Relieving the tension and tightness in the lumbar region and hips can significantly reduce this pain for the client.

Positioning for prenatal massage is not like traditional massage for obvious reasons. It is recommended that while supine, the client remains in an inclined position on the table with the knees raised up as well. To reach the client's back, she should be put in a left side-lying position with a pillow under the head and another between the legs. If there is a maternity pillow available, it can be very helpful. The maternity pillow sits on top of the massage table and allows the client to lie fully prone, since there is a hollowed space in the pillow for the client's belly. If both options are available, the massage therapist should ask the client which one they prefer.

There are many well-documented benefits of prenatal massage, but as with any modality, it is imperative that the therapist communicate with the client and obtain a full medical history. There are several possible contraindications to prenatal massage, including high risk factors, preeclampsia, severe high blood pressure, or pre-term labor. Such clients should receive clearance from their physician prior to receiving a professional massage.

Reflexology

Reflexology is based on the concept that the plantar aspect of the feet contains many pressure points that correspond to almost every part and physiological system of the body. By stimulating and releasing

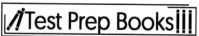

tension in these specific points, the corresponding parts of the body can become balanced and healthy. Certification in reflexology is recommended but not necessarily required, although the therapist must have excellent knowledge of the "map" of the feet to properly work the corresponding points.

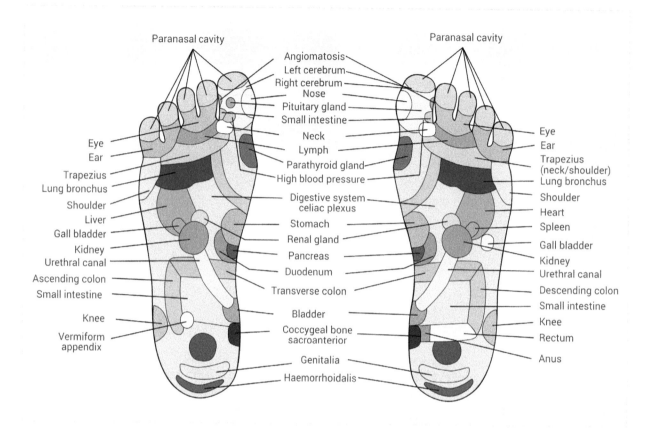

It is important to note that reflexology is not considered massage but is often lumped into the menu of massage treatments. It is common for a client to add a reflexology treatment to a massage service for an additional fee. If clients are only receiving a reflexology treatment, they may remain fully clothed, with the exception of footwear.

Contraindications for reflexology include, but are not limited to, contagious skin conditions, open wounds, viruses such as warts, sunburn, and varicose veins.

Shiatsu Massage

This modality was born out of Traditional Chinese Medicine, but the practice itself originated in Japan. Literally translated, **Shiatsu** means "finger pressure." During a Shiatsu session, the client remains fully clothed, and work is usually performed on a special floor mat. The therapists that perform this massage use a combination of pressure and stretching along what they believe to be the body's energy pathways (**meridians**). The theory of Shiatsu is that by eliminating blockages in one's **chi** (energy flow), health and wellbeing can be restored.

Contraindications for Shiatsu are bruises, inflamed skin, recent surgery, tumors, recent fractures, etc. As always, the therapist must be sure to communicate with the client regarding any health concerns that might affect the massage.

78

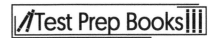

Craniosacral Therapy

Originally developed by Dr. William Sutherland and further delineated by John Upledger, D.O., in the 1970s, modern **craniosacral therapy** is a form of bodywork whereby the practitioner uses therapeutic touch to manipulate the synarthrodial joints by sensing and manipulating the subtle, rhythmic movements in living tissue. A main principle of craniosacral therapy is called "**the breath of life.**" Specially trained craniosacral therapists are able to palpate the subtle rhythms in the body known as the "**primary respiratory system.**" The benefit of this method, according to its practitioners, is that it regulates the flow of cerebrospinal fluid, which has numerous health benefits to the client.

During this treatment, the practitioner often feels a sense of being "in tune" with the client. This is called **entrainment**. It comes from lightly palpating the client's body while focusing on the body's various subtle reactions. Most clients report feeling a deep sense of relaxation after a treatment, although many of the medical benefits from craniosacral therapy have yet to be scientifically substantiated.

Oncology Massage

This modality, offered to cancer patients, is helpful in relieving stress and anxiety as well as muscle tension and fatigue that come from treatments, medications, and immobility.

If the therapy is offered in a spa setting, it gives clients a chance to relax and "escape" their disease for a short time. Being in a non-medical, serene environment goes a long way to help keep up a client's morale. If the service is offered in a hospital or hospice setting, the therapist can offer comfort and a nurturing touch in a non-invasive, non-medical way.

Certification in oncology massage is a necessity for LMTs who wish to pursue it. With oncology massage, knowing what NOT to do is just as important as knowing what to do. Getting a client's comprehensive medical history prior to any treatment is crucial. The therapist should know all of the pertinent information about a client before proceeding, such as what type of cancer the client has, whether there is a port in place, the details of blood work, the status of lymph nodes, the client's overall prognosis, and the client's level of pain on the day of treatment.

It is important to use products that are free of chemicals and fragrances and to sanitize the entire room before the oncology client arrives. This population often has compromised immunity, so keeping everything clean is crucial to the health and wellbeing of the client.

Although massage therapists are not counselors, it is not unusual for them to give words of comfort to a client dealing with life and death matters. This type of massage can be very rewarding, but it can also be stressful. The therapist will see a lot of very sick clients, some of whom may not survive. It is important for the therapist to be nurturing and caring while keeping a healthy emotional distance for their own sake.

Heat and Cold Applications

Both hot and cold therapies can help muscles heal. However, using the wrong temperature application for a particular injury can cause more damage. Generally, because of the inflammatory response, cold is used to treat acute injuries, while heat is applied for chronic issues. Cold controls the initial painful inflammatory response and gives the muscles a chance to relax as swelling goes down. Heat stimulates

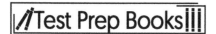

inflammation for muscles that have become locked or adhered in an uncomfortable position. In some situations, heat and cold can be used together to flush out edema.

Heat and the Inflammatory Response

When used correctly, heat therapy stimulates the inflammatory response in a hypertonic area. This reminds the brain that the area is injured, which increases blood flow, sending oxygen and nutrients to the muscles. The swelling brought on by inflammation allows the muscles to release some of their chronic tension and relax back into proper alignment. It is important not to overuse hot packs or heating pads. Because they are so comforting, many clients like to fall asleep on heating pads, which can result in serious burns. Less serious injuries can still be damaging. Too much time in a sauna, for instance, can increase inflammation to the point of unnecessary pain and swelling. A great solution for this issue is wet heat. Clients can be encouraged to take a hot bath or microwave a wet towel and apply it to the hypertonic muscle. The water will cool and evaporate naturally, making it harder to overstimulate inflammation.

Cold and Pain Relief

Cold therapy, called **cryotherapy** (such as cold packs), is used to control inflammation. This is especially useful for acute pain, such as a sprained ankle. An important acronym to remember for any acute injury is **PRICE**, which stands for **P**rotection, **R**est, **I**ce, **C**ompression, and **E**levation. To continue with the example of an injured ankle, here's how one would apply PRICE: wrap it with ace bandages (compression), and lie down with the ankle resting on pillows so it is above the level of the heart. Ice packs should be applied for 20 minutes at a time, taking 20-minute breaks in between. On occasion, the foot should be gently pronated and supinated so the ankle moves through its range of motion. If this is painful, the individual should stop moving and continue to rest.

Cold therapies will not heal the injury directly, but they relieve most pain. Indirectly, controlling inflammation prevents the body from damaging itself unnecessarily during the healing process.

Client Assessment, Reassessment, and Treatment

Organization of a Massage/Bodywork Session

A massage/bodywork session generally consists of the following steps: client consultation and evaluation (verbal intake as well as health history paperwork), written data collection, visual assessment (both general and postural), palpation assessment, range of motion assessment, and clinical reasoning (ruling out contraindications, setting treatment goals with the client, evaluating the client's response to previous treatment, and formulating treatment strategy going forward).

While this may sound overwhelming and take some time to become routine, such a work flow eventually becomes second nature.

Client Consultation and Evaluation

The front desk receptionist will generally give the client a **health history form** to complete while they wait, much like one given to a patient at a doctor's office. On this form, the client may indicate their preference for a male or female therapist, the type of service they are seeking (i.e., whether they need specific clinical work or just want to relax), the level of pressure they feel most comfortable with, and where they are experiencing pain. Clients will also include information about their medical history, such as health conditions or past surgeries that could contraindicate work on certain areas. Some massage businesses require their therapists to maintain **SOAP** (subjective, objective, assessment and plan) notes. If these are available, they can serve as a handy reference to a returning client's needs.

81

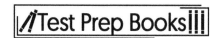

The massage therapist should consult these forms before greeting the client and leading them to the treatment room. This paperwork may help determine the questions the massage therapist asks during the **verbal intake** portion of the session, during which the therapist and client determine what issues the client is encountering and what to focus on in the session.

Often, clients don't understand the difference between a Swedish massage, in which lighter, more superficial techniques like **effleurage** (gliding) and **petrissage** (kneading) are used to induce relaxation, and deep-tissue massage, which is more clinical and targets specific areas of pain and restricted range of motion. Deep tissue massage utilizes more intense pressure and techniques like **cross-fiber friction**, in which the therapist presses into muscle fibers, rubbing perpendicular to the grain. Friction is necessary to really break up adhesions. Commonly known as knots, **adhesions** are bands of muscle fibers that stick together as a result of injury. Because friction involves sinking deep into the tissue, it is important to start with techniques like effleurage and petrissage to restore circulation to the tight, adhered muscle fibers, relaxing and softening them. Hydrotherapy with warm towels can also help prepare tissue for deeper work that may otherwise be ineffective and painful.

Adhesions don't form only as a result of a specific injury. Over time, poor posture weakens certain muscles and leads others to compensate. For example, **forward head posture**, often seen in students or people with office jobs who spend most of their day hunched over a computer, damages the erector spinae group running vertically along the length of the spine. Forward head posture forces the erector spinae to support the weight of the head, weakening the neck and causing these muscle fibers to shorten and become **hypertonic.** The body may treat this chronic stress similarly to a site of acute injury by forming scar tissue, which restricts mobility.

Hypertonic tissues possess excessive muscle tone due to tension and over-excitability of **spindle fibers**. They are more prone to painful spasms. Muscle spindles are sensory receptors within a muscle that send messages to the nervous system about that muscle's length and tension, protecting the muscle against excessive stretch.

Just as deep-tissue massage can be an intense experience for the client, causing systemic changes within the body and resulting in soreness, it demands a lot of the massage therapist physically and, as a result, is usually priced higher than a general Swedish relaxation massage.

The best way to gauge whether a client has selected the right kind of massage and understands the type of service they will receive is for the therapist to ask what level of pressure the client tends to prefer in a massage during the intake. If the client booked a Swedish massage but says they prefer deep pressure, it is helpful to explain the difference between relaxation and deep-tissue massage and ask if they would like to upgrade. The therapist should not feel obligated to perform a more tiring procedure without proper compensation. Providing excellent customer service is important, but so is self-care, especially if the therapist hopes to stay in the massage field for a long time.

Likewise, if an athlete books a Swedish massage but complains of a pulled or cramping muscle, the therapist can suggest a sports massage as a better course of treatment, as compressions and stretching alleviate strain more effectively than relaxation techniques. **Compression** includes pressing into muscles, either along or against the direction of the fibers with an open palm or closed fist, taking care not to overuse the knuckles. Although compressions are usually rhythmic and faster-paced, it is important to maintain engagement with the tissue while maintaining a steady tempo.

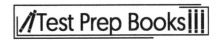

Muscle Energy Technique, or MET, is a form of stretching tailored to athletes to optimize performance and facilitate post-event recovery. The massage therapist stretches the muscle being targeted to its endpoint (as determined by asking the client when they feel pain and/or resistance) for ten seconds. Then the client contracts that same muscle against resistance by pushing against the massage therapist's hand or leg using ten to twenty percent of their full strength. The massage therapist should not push back but simply maintain their position. After approximately six seconds, the client is asked to relax so the massage therapist can repeat the passive stretching exercise. Usually, the muscle is more limber after *isometric contraction* (muscle contraction involving passive resistance, in which the muscle length does not change) and able to stretch further than before.

Proprioception is the body's sense of limb position and orientation in space. **Proprioceptors** (muscle spindles, Golgi tendon organs, and joint capsules) are special sensory organs of the nervous system that help the muscles, tendons, and joints provide information to the brain about muscle fiber and tendon tension and length, pressure, and joint angle position. Massage corrects faulty or maladaptive proprioception, communicating to the nervous system that the muscles around a site of previous injury need to be freed up instead of guarded in order to heal. It also helps facilitate relaxation of any compensating muscle groups so that proper muscle function can be restored. Muscle energy technique, in particular, helps to expand and correct proprioception. While assisted stretching may not seem as exciting or dynamic as working out an adhesion via deep friction techniques, it is actually an incredible opportunity to help someone feel freer in their body.

For returning clients, it is appropriate to inquire about the impact of previous treatments as well as their self-care regimen. The therapist should ask the client whether they have experienced decreased pain, slept more soundly, or noticed increased range of motion. A **self-care regimen** can include exercises assigned by the therapist (covered later in this guide) along with regular consumption of water, a steady exercise routine, proper nutrition, and plenty of sleep. Consistent hydration is especially important for athletes, as it helps to prevent cramping and muscle spasms, which can be extremely painful and interfere with sleep.

When a client specifies an area they would like to focus on during the session, it is important to clarify whether their pain is acute or chronic. **Acute pain** is generally the result of injury or intense strain over a short period of time. An athlete with sore muscles from over-exerting themselves or a student with neck and shoulder pain after a bout of studying, suffers from acute pain. Left untreated, acute pain resulting from injury or strain may develop into chronic pain. Repetitive stress can result in issues like tendinitis (common in violinists and other string players) and carpal tunnel syndrome (often suffered as a consequence of typing frequently). **Chronic pain** is usually defined as pain lasting six months or longer. Chronic pain may also indicate an underlying condition or disease.

Psychological conditions like anxiety and depression can interfere with how pain signals are delivered to and interpreted by the brain, even increasing their transmission. Depression is believed to be a potential cause of **fibromyalgia**, a condition involving systemic pain, near-constant fatigue, and muscle tenderness. Massage therapists should be aware of their client's holistic health, as emotional issues have biochemical, physical origins. As with depression and anxiety, those who struggle with fibromyalgia respond well to a steady sleep schedule, improved nutrition, a healthy amount of exercise, as well as regular massage treatments.

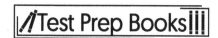

Written Data Collection

The information the client shares during verbal intake should be recorded in the **subjective** section of their SOAP note. This can include their health concerns (for example, they may complain of headaches, chronic pain, or insomnia) and priorities for the session. This can also include activities that exacerbate pain or areas of impaired functioning, such as difficulty walking up stairs or reaching kitchen cabinets.

Under the **objective** heading, the massage therapist describes the tests and assessment of the client's posture, gait, and range of motion, as well as any observations regarding muscle guarding or adhesions located during palpation.

The **activity** section details the performed procedures as well as the treatment outcome. If there is a marked improvement in circulation (indicated by warmth and tissue flushing pink or red), loosening of an adhesion, or increased range of motion—or, conversely, if the client's muscles and fasciae resist these changes—this is the place to make note of it.

Finally, the massage therapist should outline the **plan** they devise with their client for continuing care, including any assigned stretches or self-care exercises.

Visual Assessment

While massage therapists must stay within their scope of practice and not function as mental health professionals, it is important to be sensitive to a client's verbal and non-verbal cues and gauge general wellness. A highly anxious client may require more compressions, rocking, and long, soothing effleurage strokes before they relax enough to allow for deeper work. It is usually good practice to begin with deep breathing and slow, gentle touch when massaging any client, particularly one who suffers from a high degree of stress. Starting with deep pressure may only cause them to tense up more, further entrenching patterns of muscle guarding.

Analyzing **posture** and **gait** also enables the massage therapist to better tailor the session to the client's needs. The client's anterior, posterior, and lateral posture can be assessed using landmarks such as the ears, clavicles, hands, and pelvis, which ideally should be level. In a client affected by scoliosis or who tends to distribute weight to one side, one ear or shoulder may be higher than the other. The arches of the feet should also be even, resulting in equal levels of anatomic landmarks on both legs, including the popliteal fossae, patellae, and iliac crests. Any deviation of the spine or sternum from the **mid-sagittal line** may indicate postural issues and/or **scoliosis**, a condition in which mild to severe spinal curvature causes muscle imbalance, weakening certain muscles, while overburdening others.

Remember, there are three planes of the body: **sagittal, coronal** (or **frontal**), and **transverse**. The **sagittal plane** divides the body into right and left. The **mid-sagittal line** is the body's midline. All other sagittal lines run parallel to it. The **coronal plane** divides the body into anterior and posterior, while the **transverse plane** (also called the **horizontal, axial,** or **mid-axial plane**) divides the body into upper and lower halves. These reference points are incredibly useful when evaluating posture based on the placement of landmarks.

During lateral postural assessment, the massage therapist may notice that the head and neck protrude forward, past the vertical reference line, which starts just in front of the client's outer ankle. This rounding, known as **kyphosis**, is a common issue due to the amount of time people typically spend bent over a computer; clients with office jobs are especially vulnerable. Kyphosis compromises the erector

84

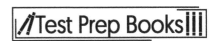

spinae muscles, which are forced to do the work of supporting the head's weight, causing pain in the upper and lower back.

Because forward head posture can lead to the development of a **dowager's hump**, the sometimes-debilitating stoop often seen in older people, it is important for the massage therapist to help clients reverse kyphosis early through self-care exercises and regular massage to prevent impaired functioning later in life. **Bruegger's relief position** is an excellent antidote to kyphotic posture. The chin is pressed toward the chest, stretching the back of the neck, and the shoulders are rolled back with the palms facing up.

The massage therapist may also notice an anterior tilt in the client's pelvis called **lordosis** or, more popularly, "**swayback**." Like kyphosis, lordosis tightens the lower back muscles and weakens the abdominals and hamstrings. Clients with a lordotic posture should be encouraged to develop an exercise routine that strengthens their core muscles in order to restore healthy pelvic alignment. **Bridges**, in which the glutes are contracted and raised while supine with knees bent, are a particularly useful core-strengthening exercise. Pilate's classes can also be helpful.

In addition to noting whether landmarks such as the ears, clavicles, and pelvis are level, the sternum should be flush with the mid-sagittal line and the hands should face medially. If the palms face outward, the client's shoulders are likely rotated, elongating the rhomboids and shortening the pectoral muscles. The midline of the client's knee joints should fall along the vertical reference line, displaying healthy alignment. Hyperextension or slight knee flexion, particularly unilaterally, may indicate past injury.

A client's gait also provides clues as to postural misalignment and resulting muscle imbalances. The massage therapist can ask clients to walk in a straight line to observe whether their knees flex equally and their feet are positioned properly without pronation or supination (indicated by the ankles rolling inward or outward). If a female client is pigeon-toed, it may be due to high heels, which can cause shortening of the gastrocnemius and soleus muscles in the calf.

Other gait deviations that may be observed during the visual assessment include:

- A client with an injured foot, ankle, knee, or pelvis may guard the compromised area, heavily favoring one side over the other, in what is known as an **antalgic gait**. To lessen pain, these clients bear most of their weight on the unaffected leg so that the stance phase is longer on the uninjured side. (The **stance phase** refers to when the foot is making contact with the ground, as opposed to the **swing phase** when the leg and foot are in the air.) An antalgic gait is also marked by a slower walking pace—less than the average of 90 to 120 steps per minute.

- An **ataxic gait** may indicate neurological problems. A client with an ataxic gait may stagger or weave, their movements jerky due to lack of balance, sensation, and poor muscle coordination caused by issues with the cerebellum. The **cerebellum** is the part of the brain in charge of balance and muscle coordination. An ataxic gait can also be caused by drinking alcohol. If a massage therapist suspects that their client may be under the influence of drugs or alcohol during the intake portion of the massage appointment, they should inform their supervisor, as intoxication is an absolute contraindication to massage therapy.

- Older clients are especially prone to displaying an **arthrogenic gait**, which is often caused by osteoarthritis or rheumatoid arthritis in the hip, knee, or ankle joints. Elevation of the pelvis on the impacted side is a clue that the client suffers from stiffness; this compensation allows for the

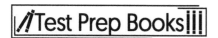
toes to clear the ground despite painful and immobile joints. In order to clear the ground, the client may lift their entire leg and have a shortened step length.

- **Trendelenburg gait** is caused by a weak or misfiring **gluteus medius**, a muscle that attaches to the **iliac crest** (upper ridge of the posterior pelvis) and sits above the glutes. It can be detected by **Trendelenburg's sign**, in which the hip drops down on the affected side during stance phase.

- A **lurching gait,** causing the client to pitch forward, is due to weakness in the glutes.

- Clients suffering from Parkinson's disease may take short, shuffling steps to compensate for lack of stability.

- A spasm in the *psoas*, a muscle that runs from the **lumbar** (lower) vertebrae to the anterior pelvis, can cause a pronounced limp. A client with **psoatic limp gait** may appear bent at the waist because the contraction of the psoas causes hip flexion. The hip may also be laterally rotated, or turned out.

- Short, tight **hip adductors**, which are the muscles responsible for pulling the thighs in toward each other, can cause a person to cross one leg in front of the other as if on a catwalk. Those with **scissors gait** typically suffer from painful muscle spasms in their upper inner thighs. This gait deviation is particularly prevalent in those with cerebral palsy.

- **Steppage gait** is due to weakness in the **dorsiflexors,** the muscles in the front of the shin that lift the toes toward the sky. It can be easily confused with arthrogenic gait because clients with this imbalance may also have an elevated pelvis on the compromised side in order to allow their toes to clear the ground. One clue to help the massage therapist distinguish between them is that a client with steppage gait may demonstrate **drop foot** when the heel strikes the ground in stance phase.

  Those with **drop foot** (also called **foot slap**) struggle to lift the front part of the foot (toe section), which consequently drags on the ground while walking. Drop foot signals larger neurological and/or muscular issues, including damage to the sciatic or peroneal nerves and muscle paralysis in the anterior compartment of the lower leg. Massaging the dorsal extensor muscles in the feet and toes (tibialis anterior, extensor digitorum longus, and extensor hallucis longus), which impinge on the peroneal nerve when tight, may alleviate drop foot. The **peroneal nerve** is the lower branch of the **sciatic nerve**, which runs from the lower back through the back of the thigh and down the lateral shins.

- A client with **hemiplegic gait** is paralyzed on one side of the body, most likely due to a **cerebrovascular incident** (commonly known as a **stroke**). On the compromised side, the shoulders will be internally rotated, the elbow and wrist will be flexed, the hip will be flexed and adducted (causing a stoop and shuffle), and the knee will be flexed.

- Joint problems or long periods of immobilization (for example, post-surgery recovery) cause muscle **contracture**, which can make walking more difficult.

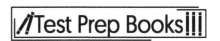

Palpation Assessment

Generally speaking, massage therapy sessions begin with the client in the **prone** position (lying on their stomach with their face in the face-cradle) under the sheet, although a therapist may choose to start in **supine** (facing up) position depending on the client's needs and what areas of the body most need addressing. After verbal intake and gait assessment, the therapist will step out of the room while the client undresses to their comfort level and knock before coming back in. Proper draping is essential for creating professional boundaries and fostering a sense of security and trust with the client, who may feel vulnerable. This means keeping the client's body covered by a sheet and only uncovering the area currently being worked on. It is appropriate for the therapist to ask if he or she may tuck the sheet into the client's underwear in order to form a clean line when undraping the back and legs. Once the area of the body being treated has been properly undraped, the therapist can proceed with assessing the condition of muscle tissue and fascia via palpation.

The goal of **palpation** assessment is to determine the health of fascia and muscle. Temperature, texture, movement, and rhythm all serve as measures of whether tissue is healthy. Muscles receiving adequate blood flow feel warm to the touch, while tissue that does not heat up or redden, even with massage, may be ischemic. **Ischemia** refers to a restriction in blood supply. Healthy muscles will also feel smooth and yielding, without adhesions or trigger points, and reasonable application of pressure will not cause the client to complain of tenderness.

Trigger points feel like pebbles beneath the surface of the skin. These adhesions in muscle and **fascia** (fibrous connective tissue between muscles and organs) refer pain to other parts of the body when pressure is applied. **Trigger point therapy** involves applying sustained pressure to these adhesions until local and referred sensation gradually diminishes. Releasing trigger points improves the health of muscle tissues.

To determine the condition of a specific muscle, it is best to locate the origin and insertion points so as to palpate the muscle's entire length. This can be done while performing range of motion exercises, such as assisted stretching, to assess the muscle's texture when contracted and slack. Limited range of motion indicates hypertonicity in muscle tissue.

It is also important to monitor the client's breathing. The human nervous system can be divided into the sympathetic and parasympathetic divisions. The **sympathetic nervous system** is responsible for the fight-or-flight response, giving the body the adrenaline necessary for a rabbit to outrun a coyote or a student to make it through a stressful exam. While under sympathetic control, the body releases high levels of cortisol, impeding the ability to breathe deeply or digest properly. Breathing and digestion are both autonomic functions—the duty of the **parasympathetic nervous system**. The job of the massage therapist is to coax clients into the relaxed state in which the body can heal itself, instead of diverting energy toward bracing itself for the next stressful ordeal. The therapist should listen for a slow, steady rhythm in the client's breathing and watch for involuntary muscle twitches. Flatulence can also be a good sign that the client's parasympathetic nervous system is taking over.

Range of Motion Assessment

During an **active range of motion assessment**, the client moves their joints themselves, stopping when they experience resistance and/or pain.

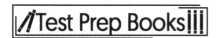
During a **passive range of motion assessment**, the massage therapist stretches the client, often past the point where the client themselves might stop. While passive range of motion assessment can help determine the client's actual level of flexibility, as opposed to their comfort zone, it is crucial to pay attention to non-verbal cues such as wincing or rapid breathing, verbal expressions of pain, and where the tissue itself offers resistance, so that no injury or strain occurs.

Clinical Reasoning

Ability to Rule Out Contraindications

Massage therapists can rule out certain contraindications visually, such as **edema** (swelling), **contusion** or **hematoma** (bruising), and **varicose veins** (the swelling of veins, causing them to be visible below or protrude from the skin). Massage therapy, particularly lymphatic drainage massage, is often appropriate and helpful in cases of edema, helping to flush out tissue and reduce fluid retention. **Pitted edema**, however, may indicate a serious cardiovascular condition or kidney dysfunction. If swollen tissue retains an indentation when pressed, the heart may not be circulating properly to the area, and massage could endanger the client. In the case of pitted edema, the client's physician should be consulted before proceeding.

Contusions and hematomas are formed when an injury causes small blood vessels to break and clots to assemble beneath the skin. Massage should be avoided in bruised areas because it will increase internal bleeding and slow healing. Varicose veins are commonly found in the legs or feet; smaller varicose veins are often referred to as spider veins. They can be harmless but can also cause aching and indicate more serious circulatory problems, such as the risk of blood clots. People who must stand for prolonged periods of time are more prone to developing varicose veins, due to the pressure this exerts on the vascular system. Some massage therapists still work on areas with varicose and spider veins using light, superficial Swedish strokes, but the risk of **embolism** (a fatal blood clot) means massage is generally contraindicated.

Because a client may not disclose important information or be aware of a health condition, it is important for massage therapists to obtain professional insurance in case they are held liable for injury. **ABMP** (Associated Bodywork and Massage Professionals) and **AMTA** (American Massage Therapy Association) are the most common providers.

Client Treatment Goal Setting

Before and after treatment, the massage therapist and client should set goals. A client complaining of shoulder pain may seek massage therapy with the goal of managing that pain. The massage therapist can evaluate the client's response to previous treatment by asking the client about changes they have noticed in their condition and by looking for increased range of motion and/or decreased hypertonicity during the session.

Formulation of Treatment Strategy

Together, the massage therapist and client should formulate a treatment strategy, deciding which techniques (Swedish, deep tissue, trigger point therapy, sports massage, hydrotherapy, etc.) will best target the client's areas of concern as well as the number and frequency of sessions necessary to properly address the issue. The massage therapist may also assign self-care exercises like Bruegger's Relief Position, positive rest position, wall angels, or IT band foam rolling. It is appropriate to advise the

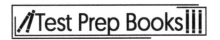

client on the benefits of a healthy lifestyle involving daily hydration, adequate sleep, good nutrition, and regular exercise.

Bruegger's Relief Position helps correct forward head posture and medial rotation of the shoulders, providing relief to the erector spinae, the trapezius muscles, and the rhomboids. If a client works at a computer all day and finds himself slouching, this exercise, easily performed at a desk, can help reverse that slump. Sitting on the edge of their chair with legs open, the client will tilt the pelvis forward, lift the chest so that the spine curves, and roll the shoulders backward with palms facing up. The chin is pressed down to the chest to stretch the erector spinae and other muscles in the back of the neck. Bruegger's Relief Position can be performed periodically throughout the day as a micro-break for maximum effectiveness.

Positive rest position stretches the erector spinae from its origin in the iliac crest (the top of the posterior pelvis) to its insertion in the cervical vertebrae, relieving pain in the neck and low and mid back. It is a very simple exercise to perform: While lying supine on the floor, the glutes are pressed against the wall with legs raised so the body forms a 90-degree angle or L shape.

Wall angels are an exercise specifically geared toward correcting medial rotation of the shoulders, offering relief to the rhomboids and pectoral muscles. Standing with back and arms flush against the wall, the client brings their elbows as close to their sides as possible without lifting their arms off the wall.

The **IT band**, or the **iliotibial tract**, is a long strip of connective tissue on the lateral thigh that runs from the iliac crest to the tibia. It frequently becomes inflamed in runners and cyclists, causing knee pain and dysfunction. Massage therapists can recommend that clients with IT band syndrome use a foam roller, but they should also advise them not to overdo it. Foam rolling can work out adhesions in the iliotibial band, but there is a point of diminishing returns, at which already overly elongated tissue is just receiving more stress.

Tension in the IT band often results from muscle imbalance. The **gluteus medius**, a muscle in the upper buttocks responsible for hip abduction (lateral or side movement), is supposed to fire during locomotion so the knee is stabilized and the patella does not slip out of position. When the gluteus medius is weak or does not fire properly, the iliotibial band is forced to do the work of stabilizing the knee joint. Clients with knee pain or tight IT bands should be encouraged to strengthen their gluteus medius as well as use a foam roller.

The gluteus medius can be strengthened by lying on one's side in the fetal position and lifting the knee while keeping the feet together, making sure that the movement originates in the hip rather than the outer thigh. The client can check by keeping their hand on their hip, near the iliac crest, to feel the gluteus medius contract. It is also important not to roll backward or forward while performing this exercise, but rather to maintain equilibrium, with the hips neatly stacked atop each other.

Ethics, Boundaries, Laws & Regulations

Ethical Behavior

Ethics are essentially rules for good behavior. Although good ethics should be a factor in any career, the fact that massage therapy deals with sensitive health issues makes ethical conduct much more important in this field. Some general aspects of good ethical behavior include therapists representing themselves truthfully and honestly to clients, not doing any harm to clients, and conveying a passion for the field of work. Other aspects are more specific to massage therapy, such as safeguarding the client's confidentiality, providing draping in a safe and comfortable manner for the client, and refusing to accept any gifts intended to influence a referral, decision, or treatment. These and other ethical behavior guidelines can be reviewed on the websites of the National Certification Board for Therapeutic Massage & Bodywork (NCBTMB) and the American Massage Therapy Association (AMTA).

Professional Boundaries

Clients get massages for a variety of reasons. In addition to having muscle tension relieved, they seek massage therapy for the experience of human touch, to relax and escape from emotional stress, and to vent to someone about their problems while receiving a relaxing massage. Because of this aspect of the business, it's easy for clients to become attached to their massage therapists and vice versa. It is encouraged for therapists to build rapport with regular clients, but they should be careful not to cross any ethical lines.

Massage therapy is a caring and nurturing business that requires a great deal of empathy and compassion, which can make it difficult to maintain clear professional boundaries. It is natural to develop strong feelings about a client after hours of conversation; caring about a person's wellbeing is truly part of an LMT's job. However, therapists cross a line if they ever become involved with the client's personal life beyond the conversations they have in-session.

It is natural for clients to develop feelings for therapists, especially when they think of their therapist as someone who is helping them through physical and emotional difficulties. Most clients are able to maintain professional boundaries with their massage therapists, but it is important for a therapist to be aware of the signs that someone is attempting to cross that line.

There are a few key steps for therapists to take to convey the message that he or she takes the issue of professional boundaries seriously and that clients are expected to maintain them as well:

- A therapist should not volunteer personal details. If a therapist is self-employed, clients might have access to the therapist's cell phone and email address to schedule appointments. It is recommended that the therapist set up separate contact information exclusively for client use; this will establish a separation between personal and professional environments.

- Self-employed therapists should not work in their personal living spaces. If one must work within the home, it is important to make sure all state licensure laws are being obeyed and that there is a separately designated area, preferably with a separate entrance. It should never be a bedroom or be within the therapist's personal living quarters.

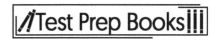

- Although it is common for clients to talk about themselves and/or their problems during a massage therapy session, the therapist should not share too much about their own personal life in return. It is appropriate for the therapist to listen and respond to the client, but telling them about one's own problems is unprofessional.

- The massage therapist should keep any kind of flirting and sexual innuendos out of the conversation at all times. If clients become flirtatious, the therapist should change the subject. If clients insist or continue, the LMT should tell them that this is an inappropriate topic of discussion and that if it continues the service will be terminated.

Code of Ethics Violations

Ethics violations are taken very seriously. Client complaints can be common in this field, especially for therapists who work in spas. It is important to distinguish between legitimate therapist ethics violations, legitimate service complaints, and clients who just like to complain to get a discount or free service.

This section is only dealing with actual ethical violations. These could include treating a client rudely, not providing the service that was scheduled, gossiping about a client, trying to diagnose and treat the client, or making inappropriate advances or contact with a client. Most places of business have a protocol for filing complaints against therapists. Usually, an investigation is conducted to determine the legitimacy of the reported events, and a course of action is determined based on the facility's policies. The following examples look at several ethical issues:

- A therapist takes a client back for service 10 minutes past the prearranged start time, even though the client was there on time. The client expresses that his neck is particularly sore, and requests extra attention in that area. Ignoring that request, the therapist spends little time on the client's neck and concludes the service at the regular finish time, effectively cutting the client's service by 10 minutes. The client is aware of this and not happy so he reports the therapist to the manager at the desk. The client is given a discount on the service just received, and the manager has a talk with the therapist. This behavior is ethically unsound because the massage therapist did not keep their promise to uphold the standard of providing the highest quality of service to the client.

- During a massage, a therapist inappropriately touches the client and makes a crude sexual comment. (The gender of either party is irrelevant here.) The client becomes physically and emotionally distraught and asks the therapist to leave the room immediately. She instantly reports the incident to the manager, at which point the manager is obligated to call the police. This behavior is highly unethical, and it jeopardizes not just the therapist's career, but also the public perception of the entire massage community. There are no warnings for this kind of behavior. This would result in the therapist's immediate termination and the loss of a license to practice massage.

- A client exits the massage studio and is relaxing in the lounge area when she overhears her therapist talking to another employee and making a derogatory comment about her. This is a clear violation of confidentiality. It is common for therapists to discuss clients with each other to share techniques or answer questions about how to treat a certain condition. However, gossiping or making fun of a client is strictly forbidden, whether or not it is within earshot of a client. This is especially important because so many clients reveal very personal details to their

91

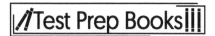

therapists, so maintaining that confidence is essential for establishing rapport with clients and employers alike.

It is important to note that most places of business have a disciplinary policy regarding reprimands, both verbal and written. It is up to the therapist to be aware of their employer's proper conduct policies as explained in the employee manual.

The Therapeutic Relationship

The therapeutic relationship is a delicate one. Clients exhibit a great deal of trust in their therapists: they are undressed, they allow someone to touch their body in new ways, and they agree to follow the directions of someone with whom they are not personally acquainted. This is a very vulnerable position to be in. The client needs to have a certain amount of faith in the therapist's abilities as a practitioner and as a compassionate person. Clients must trust that their therapists cannot only help them heal, but also respect their dignity and privacy.

There is a power differential between client and therapist. It is common for a client who feels positive results from massage therapy sessions to project a certain amount of power onto the massage therapist as someone who has the knowledge and skills to solve the client's problems. It is important for the massage therapist to acknowledge this power dynamic and never take advantage of the situation.

Often, a client will mistake the therapist's bodywork skills for the ability to diagnose conditions. It is crucial that therapists work exclusively within their scope of practice and not diagnose or treat medical conditions. Certain muscular issues can obviously be evaluated by a massage therapist, but if a herniated disc is suspected, for example, it is best to suggest that the client see a doctor for a proper diagnosis.

Maintaining a long-term relationship with a client takes effort and insight. Staying in tune with a client's physical and emotional health requires some intuitive talent and a great deal of care. Maintaining an open line of communication is key to keeping a healthy therapeutic relationship and long-term client.

Dual Relationships

Almost every therapist will face several dual relationships over the course of a career and this is a tricky part of the business. A **dual relationship** is where the client is not just a client; they might also be a relative, friend, or business associate. These relationships can be very sensitive. If not handled professionally, they can cause some serious problems.

Massage therapy is in high demand. From the moment an aspiring therapist starts school, friends and relatives will most likely ask for services. In these cases, it is important to maintain professional boundaries when in a therapeutic setting. It is important to designate a massage space and to treat these people like any other clients, as this will help maintain mutual respect.

An important distinction to be made with dual relationships is the order in which the two relationships began. Did the therapist meet the client before or after starting treatment? If they were friends first, the therapist should draw clear lines, especially when it comes to charging for services. Sometimes people close to the therapist will expect to receive services for free. The therapist needs to be careful in situations such as this, since once a precedent is set, it will be hard to break. If the therapist agrees to give free massages initially, then this will continue to be expected. Spouses and partners are exceptions

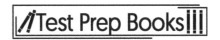

to this dual relationship issue; however, hopefully those people in the therapist's life will not take advantage.

It is important for therapists to remember that massage is their livelihood. Just like any other profession, such as doctor, chef, or electrician, there is a time when it is fine to take a break. An electrician does not want to go to a party and be asked to fix a wiring problem. A doctor does not want to go out to dinner with friends and be bombarded with medical questions. The same goes for a massage therapist, who should not feel obligated to fix friends' physical problems at every social event.

The dual relationships that occur with clients after they become clients are the ones that really raise a caution flag. Deciding to take a therapist-client relationship outside of the office is one that must be carefully thought through and is usually inadvisable.

First, the therapist must be conscious of transference and countertransference. **Transference** is when a client develops feelings toward the therapist that are similar to feelings he or she might have for someone outside of that professional relationship. For example, a client going through a divorce may develop romantic feelings for the therapist if massage is the client's only consistent way of experiencing touch. These feelings are understandable but should not be acted upon.

Countertransference occurs when the therapist develops inappropriate feelings toward the client. When this happens, the therapist might engage in personal conversations with the client or have a desire to socialize with that person outside the office setting. For example, after learning during a massage therapy session that the client shares the same passion for wine that the therapist does, the therapist may invite the client to a wine tasting.

These might seem like harmless situations, and as long as neither party acts on their feelings, that is generally true. Most therapists will experience some sort of transference, countertransference, and dual relationship issues over the course of their careers. Misplaced feelings can result in unrealistic expectations and can damage a person's career as a result.

Many therapists barter their services with clients. This can be a win-win situation, but as always, it must be approached carefully. Goods and services exchanged should be of equal value, otherwise both parties risk resentment. Bartering should also take place in a reasonable time frame; a therapist shouldn't offer her services in January and expect to be paid in July. Just as in any dual relationship, there must be clear communication, either verbally or in writing, about what goods or services are being bartered.

The riskiest dual relationship is when a therapist and a client become romantically involved. This is slightly different from sexual misconduct, which will be described below. Even so, this behavior is strongly discouraged. If a therapist meets a person as a client and the two of them decide to begin a romantic relationship, they must cease their professional relationship before they can legally date.

It is not uncommon for either a massage therapist or a client to feel either an emotional or physical attraction to the other. However, the people involved should be absolutely sure that their feelings are genuine and not the result of transference. Massage therapy is very physically intimate, even at its most clinical level, and it can inspire many emotions. If the attraction stems from transference, projection, or convenience, it must be dismissed immediately. It is best to terminate the relationship entirely and refer the client to another therapist.

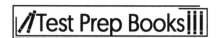

However, if each party feels a genuine (and above all, **mutual**) attraction, then it must be addressed in a serious and professional manner. Once both adults consent, the professional relationship must end immediately. It is unethical for a therapist to date a client (although it can be ethical to offer massage to a partner outside a professional setting).

Sexual Misconduct

There is absolutely no tolerance for any kind of sexual misconduct in massage therapy. This applies to therapists and clients alike. If either party makes an unsolicited sexual advance, the relationship should be immediately terminated and the offending party dismissed from the practice.

The massage therapy industry still has to battle misconceptions about sexual behavior, and any attempt to use clinical massage for sexual release only supports that image. **Massage therapy** is medically-based and requires intense medical and clinical training. It is not sex work. Terms such as masseuse, massage parlor, and massage bed (as opposed to "massage table") should never be used. It is perfectly acceptable to correct other people's use of these damaging terms.

A therapist who commits an act of sexual misconduct will face severe professional and legal consequences. More often, however, the therapist must protect herself or himself (socially, professionally, and even sometimes physically) from amorous clients. It is important for the therapist to have a plan for how to deal with these situations, should they arise.

There are varying degrees of sexual misconduct. Although none of them are acceptable, there are various ways to handle different situations. If a client makes a casual off-color comment or exhibits physical arousal during the massage, the therapist should respond as quickly and tactfully as possible by redirecting the conversation. For example, during a massage, a client might make a comment to the therapist such as, "I'll bet your husband must love your massages." This is usually a probing question to find out if the therapist is married, but it is inappropriate nonetheless. A good response for the therapist to give is, "I'm sorry, but I don't discuss my personal life with my clients," or, "Yes, he does." Whether the therapist is married or not, it usually ends that line of discussion.

If a client goes even further over the line by attempting to grab the therapist, making an overtly sexual comment, or asking for a sexual service during the massage, then the therapist must immediately terminate the service, leave the room, and get back-up. It is ideal to speak to a manager, but a self-employed therapist might need to get their receptionist or even call a friend. The client should be escorted off the premises immediately. Should the therapist so choose, the legal authorities can be called in.

If the therapist is the perpetrator of sexual misconduct, she risks losing her license. When a massage therapist violates the ethics of the profession, it reflects poorly on all therapists and serves to further perpetrate false perceptions.

Instances of sexual misconduct on the part of the massage therapist could include flirting, giving out personal information for the purpose of dating or having a sexual encounter, or performing any kind of sexual act during a massage therapy service. All of these behaviors are unacceptable in the field.

Working at a spa in a hotel or casino increases the likelihood of sexual misconduct on the client's part. The transient nature of these settings makes some people see relationships with staff as disposable. It is important for therapists in such environments to be well-prepared with verbal warnings and service

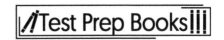

terminations in those situations. However, many therapists can work a lifetime without ever encountering such clients. Therapists should be aware of these potentially inappropriate situations without becoming too overwhelmed. The vast majority of clients are seeking massage therapy for therapeutic purposes.

Massage Bodywork-Related Laws and Regulations

Done correctly, massage therapy has positive effects on a person's health and wellbeing. Conversely, massage therapy can have an adverse effect on one's health if performed incorrectly or if the therapist is improperly educated. This can pose a safety concern for the public. For any profession that deals with public health and wellness, all parties benefit from having certain governmental protections in place.

Therefore, it is a reasonable expectation for the therapist to be properly trained, qualified, and licensed. This is beneficial to the health and safety of both the client and the therapist. Most states have rigorous certification guidelines to ensure that all legitimately operating massage therapists are working up to the same consistent standards.

Each state sets forth standards of qualifications and scope of practice guidelines to maintain a level of competency through education and standardized testing. The government establishes clear rules about a therapist's scope of practice to prevent him or her from making inaccurate and illegal diagnoses. Most states mandate that aspiring LMTs meet certain eligibility requirements to maintain licensure, including accruing continuing education units (CEUs) or classes to stay abreast of medical innovations and best practices.

State licensing boards offer therapists and businesses the means to make legislative changes; to create, mandate, and enforce disciplinary policies; and update rules and regulations that apply to all members of the field. This offers a safety net and official resource for both massage therapists and the public they serve.

It is critical for massage therapists to obtain credentials and work legally within the state(s) of their choice. State licensing is the only legal document required for an LMT. It can be obtained only after a candidate has completed education from an accredited school and passed the state licensing exam. There are usually requirements to maintain the license, such as taking a certain number of CEUs and paying annual renewal fees. It is illegal in most states to operate as a massage therapist without a state license.

Once someone has a state license, this therapist may decide to also become board-certified through the National Certification Board for Therapeutic Massage and Bodywork (NCBTMB). Although this certification is not a substitute for a state license, it does show that the therapist is further qualified through the rigorous standards set forth by this accreditation board. Achieving this credential is not legally required in order to practice, but it does add some degree of credibility.

As helpful and unifying as state laws and regulations are for massage therapists, they come with some caveats. The most challenging is that regulations are not consistent from state to state. States require different numbers of hours for certification, different requirements for maintaining a license, different fees, and different renewal policies. There are still a few states that have no regulated licensure at all. For example, Minnesota has no state licensing laws but leaves it up to individual municipalities within the state to create and enforce their own regulations. There are regulations in place under the Unlicensed Complementary and Alternative Health Care Practices Act that massage therapists are

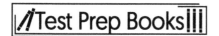

supposed to comply with. States like New Jersey, Florida, and California all require 500 hours of training by an accredited school and the passing of a state board licensing exam. New York is one of the strictest in the country, requiring aspiring massage therapists to complete 1000 hours of training in a program registered by the New York State Education Department.

These vast differences make it challenging for a massage therapist to move from state to state and continue working. Some states will take into account one's actual field experience when applying for a new state license, while others will require the therapist to go back to school if he or she has fewer education hours than what the new state requires. If a therapist plans to move across state lines, it is important to start the transfer process as early as possible. Obtaining a new license can take weeks or even months. It is possible to hold licenses in more than one state, which can be necessary for therapists who travel regularly.

Overall, statewide regulation of massage therapy works in the therapists' favor. It legitimizes businesses and protects employees, creating highly principled standards of practice. In addition to state standards and regulations, massage therapists have organizations such as the American Massage Therapy Association (AMTA), which is the largest non-profit professional association for massage therapists, students, and schools to get help navigating all of the aspects of the profession.

Scope of Practice

The **scope of practice** describes what a professional is and is not allowed to do within a work setting. All professions have a defined scope of practice, although they are often more rigorous for healthcare providers. For example, a pharmacist can dispense medications but not prescribe them, and a math teacher can teach math in the classroom but cannot show up at a child's house unannounced to make sure the child is doing homework. In massage therapy, being aware of one's scope of practice at all times is crucial for the safety of the therapist as well as the client.

Defining the scope of practice in the massage therapy industry has been challenging. As mentioned previously, one of the difficulties with state licensing is that so many states have different requirements; there is no uniformity in qualifying therapists. The same issue exists with the scope of practice. Every state has its own set of rules and some states have even outlawed certain modalities, such as medical massage or craniosacral therapy. Many regulating entities state that massage therapists cannot "treat" any ailment; but this can be an issue of semantics and how one defines "treat."

No matter where one works or lives, there are some strict cardinal rules within a massage therapist's scope of practice. First and foremost, therapists should never diagnose a client. It is common for a massage therapist with anatomical and clinical experience to detect a medical issue that a client might have, but the therapist should never diagnose the suspected problem. Instead, he or she should mention a possible concern to the client and suggest an appointment be made with an appropriate physician for an official diagnosis. For example, if a massage therapist notices a dark mole on the client's back, it is not within the therapist's scope of practice to suggest that the client probably has cancer. They should let the client know what was noticed and refer the client to their physician.

It is important for therapists not to purport to be experts in areas in which they are not. Training in new modalities should be thorough, accredited, and hands-on in order for a therapist to add it to their scope of practice.

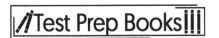

Speaking poorly about fellow professionals, including medical professionals and other massage therapists, is not only outside the scope of practice, but also in poor taste. This also includes contradicting or offering a conflicting opinion about medical advice that a client received from a doctor or another medical professional. It is not within a massage therapist's scope of practice to prescribe an anecdote. Rather, they can generally suggest or relay an anecdote that may be helpful, encouraging the client to further research the issue. For example, in the case of a client with back spasms, the therapist may be fairly confident that a series of massages will eventually correct the spasms. However, the client's doctor wants to administer cortisone shots and muscle relaxers immediately. The therapist should not contradict the doctor's recommendations, but simply state the benefits of massage therapy in this situation and perhaps suggest the client obtain a second opinion before proceeding with the doctor's recommended treatment.

A therapist's scope of practice may also be dictated by her place of business. For example, some spas may allow massage therapists to perform body treatments such as wraps or scrubs, which are clearly not massages, while other spas may only allow estheticians to offer those services. It is important for massage therapists to be aware of the scope of practice regulations within the state and town in which they work. Some states don't allow any kind of stretching, whereas others do, for example. Therefore, in addition to the general professional scope of practice guidelines discussed above, it is necessary for therapists to research their individual place of employment and place of residence to make sure that they are complying with all of the scope of practice regulations that may exist.

Professional Communication

Irish playwright George Bernard Shaw said it best: "The single biggest problem in communication is the illusion that it has taken place." It is just as important for therapists to master communication as it is for them to study massage therapy. There are various levels and dynamics of communication in the field, especially because therapists interact with such diverse clientele. There are three kinds of relationships, in particular, that a therapist will engage in repeatedly: those with clients, fellow therapists, and employers. Therapists must learn to clearly and consistently navigate communication in all three of these relationships.

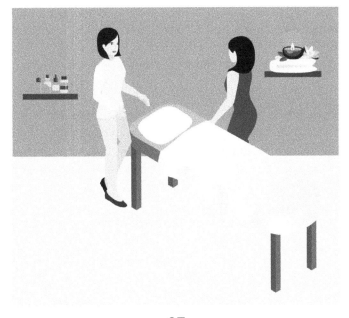

97

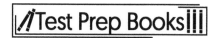

Communication between the therapist and the client is arguably the most important of these relationships. The first phase of the therapist-client relationship is the **intake**. It is imperative to allow clients to feel comfortable even before service begins. Clients should be able to communicate their issues, some of which might be personal or sensitive, and ask questions without fear of judgment. The therapist must communicate an air of accessibility to the client and must know the right questions to ask without making the client feel awkward. Thorough communication skills enable the therapist to safely and effectively help the client, while simultaneously giving the client space to relax and release some emotional tension. Maintaining eye contact and using active listening techniques and supportive verbal and non-verbal communication is imperative to building good rapport.

The second phase of communication occurs during the **service.** While it is not recommended that a therapist engage the client in conversation, it is important for the therapist to check in with the client at least twice to assess comfort level regarding such factors as pressure and temperature.

The final phase is **post-service**. Communicating with clients about how they feel and answering any new questions is crucial at this time. The therapist can also communicate any suggestions on how to maintain the benefits of the massage. This is also a great time to recommend particular stretches, or refer the client to a chiropractor or another allied health professional, if necessary.

Therapists who work with each other in spas or medical offices should communicate to ensure the clients' safety and to boost morale among the staff. Maintaining proper clinical notes is critical when multiple therapists see the same client. Verbally sharing client information pertaining to treatment or issues with other therapists is also important, as long as confidentiality is respected. For example, a therapist may have been seeing a client for therapeutic relaxation purposes, but the client has serious medical issues including a surgery several years ago, in which a shunt was placed in his brain. As a result, scalp massage and acute cervical manipulation are contraindicated for him. On a day when his regular therapist is busy, the client may come in to see another therapist. The original therapist should have a clear description of the client's medical issues listed wherever client notes are kept, and, if possible, that therapist should verbally discuss the issue with the new therapist so that the client's wellbeing is made a top priority.

Within a workplace, a veteran therapist often will mentor a newer therapist. In these situations, communication should remain open and accessible for both parties. Veteran therapists need to help newer ones, and newer ones need to listen to veteran ones. Maintaining this level of open communication and helpfulness translates to the type of positive and healing experience that clients deserve.

Finally, the way therapists and management communicate is critical to maintaining a properly staffed workplace. There should always be an open-door policy when it comes to communication, so that therapists feel comfortable addressing any issues that arise with management. It is important for management to be accessible and understanding. In particular, therapists must feel safe to communicate about their own health and capacity for taking on new clients, as well as about any controversial client issues that might arise. For instance, if a client engages in sexual misconduct with a therapist, the therapist must feel safe going to management as an authoritative and supportive resource to deal with the situation.

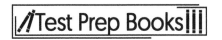

As in any relationship, personal or professional, the quality of communication will determine the health, longevity, and wellbeing of the relationship itself. This concept is at the heart of a massage therapist's purpose and mission.

Confidentiality

Confidentiality is the primary subject of a massage therapist's code of ethics. Clients reveal sensitive, personal, and medical information to their massage therapists, and it is imperative that their information remain confidential and safe. This applies to both verbal and written forms of communication.

All intake forms and chart notes should be kept in a safe place that only fellow therapists can view for clinical purposes. A locked file cabinet is a good place to keep documents of this kind. If sensitive notes are kept on a computer, access must be password-protected and shared only with authorized professionals.

Similarly, if a client verbally reveals something personal and sensitive to the therapist, it is that therapist's ethical duty to keep it confidential. The therapist can make an exception if professional advice is needed on how to proceed; however, it is best to keep the client's name private, unless it is absolutely necessary to reveal it.

Many massage therapists today wonder if they are legally required to be HIPAA-compliant. **HIPAA** stands for the Health Insurance Portability and Accountability Act. It is a law designed to keep personal health information private and secure. In the age of electronic transmissions and multiple insurance carriers, HIPAA has become necessary to help ensure patients' medical information doesn't get into the wrong hands. Most people who have visited a doctor's office in the past few years are familiar with signing a HIPAA release, stating who is approved to receive medical information on the patient's behalf.

But does this apply to massage therapists? This is a complicated question. While privacy is simply an ethical issue that should always be adhered to, the legal answer depends on the business itself. HIPAA compliance is determined by whether a business is a "covered entity." For a business to be considered a **covered entity**, it must be transmitting medical information to third-party carriers such as insurance companies. If a massage therapist works at a spa or as a sole proprietor, then he or she would not be a covered entity and, therefore, is not required to be HIPAA-compliant. If, however, a massage therapist works for a chiropractic office or physical therapy business, then claims are likely being submitted to insurance companies and HIPAA laws will apply.

Principles

The general principles of massage therapy should remain at the forefront of the massage therapist's mind. They are at the heart of the profession.

Increasing circulation is arguably the main principle and physical benefit of massage therapy. Both blood and lymphatic flow are increased during massage, bringing healing and enhancement to all of the body's physiological systems. General massage strokes should always move proximally toward the heart, to maximize the circulation benefits and keep the circulatory system functioning properly.

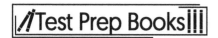

Stretching and releasing tight and adhered muscle fibers is another key principle of massage therapy and the one that most clients are seeking. The various strokes of massage, including effleurage, petrissage, and tapotement, are used to achieve this goal.

Proper body mechanics are important for any therapists who wish to maintain their physical health. Specifically, therapists should be mindful of proper posture and table height, since these techniques enable them to give an effective massage without exhausting or injuring themselves. Also, the use of correct hand and arm techniques while massaging will contribute to a massage therapist's longevity. Finally, it is best to maintain physical contact with a client as much as possible during a massage. This assures the client's sense of comfort, safety, and security during the service.

Helping to bridge the mind-body connection is a key principle of massage therapy that should be incorporated into every massage that a therapist performs. A healthy mind leads to a healthy body, and a healthy body leads to a healthy mind. Massage therapy can support the connection between the two.

The principle of stress reduction works symbiotically with the mind-body connection. Massage eases the muscle tension caused by emotional stress, so massage can release emotional tension as well. In this principle, environment is as important as the massage. Soft lighting and relaxing music help to create an atmosphere that fosters mental and emotional relaxation, allowing the physical benefits of the massage to bring the client's body back to health and wholeness.

Guidelines for Professional Practice

Proper and Safe Use of Equipment and Supplies

Massage therapists should always make time to learn about available supplies. Depending on the setting, therapists may be asked to use table warmers, hydrocollators, warming/cooling lotions, essential oils, hot stones, traction beds, exfoliating scrubs, and many other items. Knowing how to safely operate equipment and utilize the various creams and oils are extremely important. Without proper training, the therapist risks appearing unprofessional and injuring the client.

Therapist Hygiene

It is important for any healthcare provider to have excellent personal hygiene so clients are as safe and comfortable as possible. This is particularly important for massage therapists, who engage in a great deal of physical contact with clients during treatment. The guidelines for hygiene are unique in this field, given the intimate nature of massage therapy.

Scents and Essential Oils

Therapists should attend to their breath and body odor carefully and avoid any strong scents or perfumes. Many clients are sensitive to smells, and what pleases one person may give another a headache. This also applies to any essential oils or scents used in the treatment room. It is best to consult and get consent from a client before burning incense or applying essential oils to their body. Hypoallergenic lotion and scentless oil—like grapeseed or canola oils—are excellent options for the sensitive client. It is also important to ask the client about any allergies they may have, especially when using certain carrier and essential oils.

Hand Hygiene

Massage therapists must pay special attention to their hands. Hangnails or open wounds (even paper cuts) can be dangerous for the client and therapist alike. In the event of a wound, the therapist should wear a latex glove or finger cot to protect against infection. Nails must be kept short—never past the tip of the finger—and unpainted, because nail polish can harbor bacteria. Keep a nail file handy; even short nails can become ragged, potentially scratching and injuring a client.

Sanitation and Cleanliness

Massage therapists should follow standard precautions when keeping their practices clean. Standard precautions are a very specific set of guidelines designed to prevent the spread of infectious diseases. In accordance with these rules, massage therapists should:

- wash their hands thoroughly before and after working with each client.
- sanitize the work surface (the massage table) between sessions.
- cover their nose and mouth while coughing.
- avoid contact with clients' bodily fluids, including blood, mucus, semen, vaginal secretions, saliva, etc. Note that sweat is not considered an infectious bodily fluid. Contact with a client's perspiration is acceptable within these guidelines.

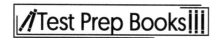

In addition to standard precautions, therapists should be diligent about laundering all cloth products. These include sheets, towels, blankets, and anything that comes into contact with a client's body. It is unacceptable to use an unwashed sheet or towel during a session. Therapists should keep extra supplies on hand at all times in case a client requests an extra sheet or towel.

Safety Practices

Facilities

All equipment should be in good working condition, and it should be tailored to suit the therapist's needs. For example, a therapist should know the table height appropriate for their own body and be aware that this height may change with different shoe styles. Also, the therapist should be cognizant of the ambiance of the room: Is it properly ventilated, or will summer heat make the client sweat uncontrollably? Is there a window? If so, does it permit people outside to look in while clients are unclothed? Are the lights on a dimmer or a switch? Who controls the music? Can anyone else in the building overhear conversations when the door is shut? Therapists should never underestimate the importance of privacy; some clients will lie about their health rather than risk being overheard by a stranger.

Whether practicing in a spa, a clinic, a hospital, or a rented room, massage therapists must prepare for all eventualities. Supplies that should be easily accessible include:

- hypoallergenic oil and lotion for clients who cannot tolerate certain chemicals.
- extra sets of clean sheets in case of spills or stains.
- pillows, bolsters, and towels for clients with limited mobility.
- cleaning supplies.
- tissues and hair ties placed in the massage room itself, so clients can use them as needed during treatment.

Therapist Personal Safety

Every massage therapist should carry professional liability insurance. This is a prerequisite of employment at most spas and clinics. Many LMTs use the insurance offered by the **American Massage Therapy Association (AMTA)**. This insurance protects against client injury and malpractice lawsuits. In addition to legal protections, massage therapists must draw clear boundaries with clients. Unfortunately, it is not uncommon for clients to seek massage in hopes of more intimacy than a therapist may legally provide. To avoid any confusion on this front, therapists should have excellent communication skills and a strong support network. Clients with amorous intentions are usually put off by the presence of a receptionist, a doctor, or even a fellow massage therapist who can assist in clear communication.

Massage therapists can also run into unique issues when dealing with clients they know and trust. For example, a massage student may be required to accrue a certain number of hours outside of class and because she is a student, she cannot be legally paid for her work, so the sessions are free. The student may have a friend who loves getting massages and agrees to receive regular massages from the therapist during school for free. When the student graduates, she begins to seek private clients, charging $100 per hour, while her friend is used to receiving the same work for free. It is easy to see how this situation could be difficult to navigate. Even more common are friends who casually seek help from well-established massage therapists. People will often approach therapists at parties or other

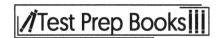
gatherings to ask for advice or hands-on work. It can be difficult to say no in these situations. Massage therapists, like most healthcare workers, want to help people and it is difficult to turn away a friend in pain. However, it is important to set clear and consistent boundaries so the therapist does not get overwhelmed by requests to work for free.

Client Safety

There are a number of steps LMTs should take to protect their clients. Proper education is of primary importance. Therapists should have practical knowledge of a wide variety of pathologies so they can accurately assess whether a client can safely receive a massage. Comprehensive insurance also ensures client safety; in the event that the therapist makes a mistake resulting in injury to the client, insurance will help resolve the issue. As the adage goes, an ounce of prevention is worth a pound of cure. Therapists should conduct thorough written and verbal intake evaluations with each new client and also make time to check in with returning clients before each treatment session. This process serves many purposes: it keeps the therapist informed about the client's health; it shows the client that the therapist is personally invested in their healing process; and it serves as a segue into treatment itself, giving both people time to connect with each other.

Therapist Care

Body Mechanics

Different massage modalities use different styles of movement, but they all have one thing in common: prioritizing the health and longevity of the massage therapist. Some tips to preserve the health of the massage therapist include the following:

Use the Correct Table Height

The surface should be at the lowest possible setting, allowing the therapist to lunge deeply and lean in toward the client as they lie supine or prone. This maximizes the amount of force a therapist can apply, even with minimal effort. Gravity does most of the work, and the therapist need not rely on their own physical strength.

Be Aware of Lines of Force

A rudimentary knowledge of physics is extremely useful, although intuition can serve just as well. In short, the therapist's limbs should extend from their core in straight lines, so the pressure is applied in a line that points directly from the center of gravity. It is incorrect, for example, to place a hand on the client's back, bend the elbow slightly, and push down with the palm. Similarly, thumbs should be held in line with the wrist at all times so the metacarpals stack on top of the carpal bones and phalanges and force is distributed evenly up the arm. This takes stress off the extremities and increases the therapist's maximum possible pressure.

Gaze Ahead

The direction of the eyes and head has a great impact on the cervical muscles. New therapists are often inclined to look down at their work, watching their hands. On rare occasions, it is important to see how a client's body reacts to the work being done. This might be true for a particularly persistent fascial restriction, for example, or an area of extreme inflammation and bruising due to acute injury. Most often, however, the information a therapist gleans from their hands is sufficient. Raising the head while

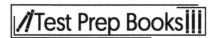
working will reduce the strain on cervical muscles and erectors and will keep the therapist's body healthy in the long term.

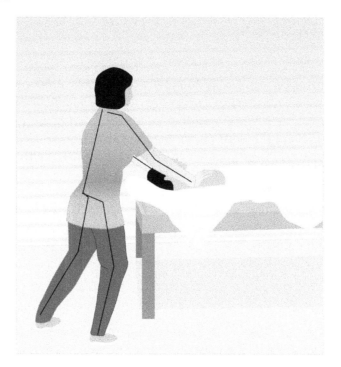

Protective Gear

Protective gear prevents infection for the client and therapist alike. Bear in mind, however, that the efficacy of this gear is limited in the profession. A therapist can only keep so much distance from a sick client until massage becomes ineffective. Masks are useful if the therapist has a cough, as they stop the spread of infected saliva and mucus; however, masks will not protect the therapist from a sick client. Gloves are the most effective barrier when either the client or therapist has open wounds, but they come with an unfortunate stigma. Working on a client while wearing latex gloves often sends the message that they are unclean and the therapist is uncomfortable or afraid of them.

This can interfere with the healing atmosphere of a massage session and make treatment less effective. **Finger cots** represent a useful middle ground; they protect the therapist without sending an upsetting message to the client. Unfortunately, finger cots are really only useful when the therapist is the injured party. It is possible to get creative with protective gear in the context of massage. Some clients prefer to receive bodywork through a layer of cloth such as a shirt, towel, or sheet. Always err on the side of caution when there is a risk of infection; it is better to cancel a massage than to spread a dangerous disease.

Self-Care

It is difficult to be an effective healer when the therapist's own body is in pain. It is vital for massage therapists to take excellent care of themselves. Massage therapists should be mindful to stretch and exercise regularly, eat well and stay hydrated, get adequate sleep, and find ways to relax outside of work, including getting massages. Generally, the therapist should take the same advice they would give to a client who has a demanding job. Successful massage therapists are highly empathetic, and it is all

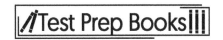

too easy to get lost in the constant flow of information received at work. To do the job well on a daily basis, the therapist must listen to other people's bodies, stresses, and worries all day, but to do their job well in the long term, therapists must find ways to turn off that empathy. Therapists should find relaxing methods of self-care and stress relief such as cooking, spending time with friends and family, gardening, yoga, and any other pursuit that helps them unwind.

Injury Prevention

Massage therapists perform bodywork to help clients alleviate stress and recover from injuries, but the work performed by massage therapists can potentially put stress on their own bodies and result in various types of injuries. There are many variables that contribute to the risk of injury, such as performing the same movements and techniques repeatedly or staying in uncomfortable positions for too long. To keep injuries from occurring, massage therapists should make sure they're using a variety of techniques, whether throughout a session or throughout a week. It's best to fluctuate between more forceful work such as deep tissue massage and more gentle techniques such as effleurage.

The positioning of the body is another important factor in preventing injury. Massage therapists should be mindful of posture and the positioning of the wrists, thumbs, elbows, neck, and head. A neutral position of the head and neck as well as the wrists can prevent issues such as muscle tension and tendonitis. The height of the massage table is also crucial in maintaining proper posture and positioning of the body. Additionally, the body of a massage therapist needs to remain strong and flexible in order to maintain certain postures and perform the techniques needed during massage sessions, therefore working out and stretching regularly are good habits that contribute to injury prevention. Massage therapists should also take time to rest between sessions.

Even seemingly minor injuries can have serious consequences for a massage therapist. If an accountant cuts her finger while slicing vegetables, there's a chance that typing will be difficult for a couple of days, however this could be more detrimental for a massage therapist. If a massage therapist sustains the same injury, he or she will likely need to take off work for a week. Activities that many people take for granted, such as cooking, cleaning, carrying heavy groceries, and using power tools, can be especially risky for massage therapists, due to potential hand injuries. Repetitive use injuries are common and can result in muscle strain over time. There has to be a balance; it is unreasonable to suggest that a massage therapist should never bake cookies for fear of burning a hand on a hot oven. At the same time, some amount of caution can go a long way. The therapist should not be afraid to ask for help and should wear gloves whenever possible; this is an extremely important part of self-care.

Draping

Safe and Appropriate

Massage sessions are a unique experience in that they require the client to be undressed and touched by a person they may have never met before. Draping is a skill that massage therapists need to master in order to make clients feel secure and relaxed. Proper draping can keep clients from feeling too exposed and relieve any tension they may have about being undressed. Although the main goal of draping is to reduce exposure of the client's body, draping also provides warmth, which aids in comfort and relaxation.

Massage therapists should learn how to cover and uncover the various areas of the body without exposing private areas while doing so. The only part of the body that should be exposed at any given time is the area that is currently being worked on by the massage therapist. As work moves to different

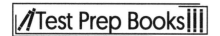
parts of the body, the massage therapist should neatly and effortlessly cover the area just worked on and uncover the next area that will be massaged. In addition to a client's privacy and security, allergies and sensitivities need to be considered. The towels or sheets that are used for draping must be clean and soft. It's best to use a detergent that is natural and does not contain scents or chemicals. Some clients are easily irritated by such ingredients.

Various bodywork modalities employ unique styles of draping. Patients in a clinic will have different expectations than vacationing swimmers at a resort or athletes at the end of a marathon. No matter the context, the therapist should make sure the draping is secure and tidy. Sheets should never be tangled or get in the way of a client's comfort or the therapist's work. Practice makes perfect; the therapist can benefit from testing new styles of draping on a friend before using them in a session.

Communication

While communication during a massage session is typically kept to a minimum, the massage therapist must be sure to communicate to the client before undraping any part of the body. This will add to the trust that is being built between the client and the massage therapist. Clients feel safer when they know ahead of time which body parts will be exposed. Communication is also made nonverbally by allowing the draping material to be a boundary between areas to be touched and areas that are not to be touched. If more of the body needs to be exposed to work on an area, the massage therapist can either inform the client of their next move in adjusting the sheet or towel or ask permission to make the adjustment.

The therapist and client should have similar goals for each session. Consent is important at every point in a massage, especially when deciding which areas to work on. Sometimes it is medically necessary to work on body parts, such as the glutes or proximal adductors, that are not touched in most professional circumstances in our culture. It is important for the therapist to communicate clearly and get the client's consent before working on these areas. Some clients will think they are being tactful when they are actually being vague. For example, some people suffering from sciatica will go to great lengths to avoid talking about glute pain, reporting, "my hips hurt" or, "my lower back hurts."

It can also be difficult for a massage therapist to assess what a client means when he or she lacks the anatomical vocabulary he needs to describe a sensation or location. In these cases, the therapist should trust their intuition and maintain a relevant conversation while working on the area in question. Questions like, "Does this hurt?" and, "Am I on the worst spot, or right next to it?" can be useful.

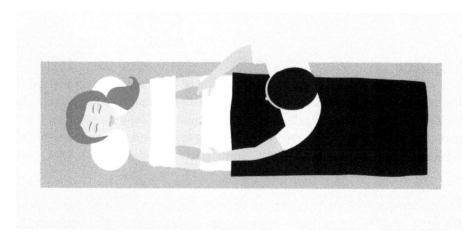

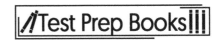
Above all, the therapist needs to respect the wishes of the client. If the therapist undrapes a client's glutes—or arms, knees, or any other structure—and the client slides the sheet back to cover the area, it is the therapist's responsibility to leave the sheet where the client placed it. Consciously or not, the client chose to send a clear message about boundaries, and this message must be respected. The therapist can try setting the tone for this level of respect at the very beginning of the session with a phrase like, "Please undress to your level of comfort." This lets the client know that they are in control of the session, and that the therapist will never touch their body in a way that makes them uncomfortable.

Business Practices

As in any business, it is important for the expectations of a clinic or spa to be clearly communicated to all employees and clients. Whether the LMT owns their own practice or works for an employer, it is important to set clear boundaries and goals before starting a new job. Some helpful questions to bear in mind when joining or starting a new practice include the following:

- How many hours per week is the therapist expected to work? Is this physically feasible?
- Who is responsible for the general maintenance of supplies (doing laundry, stocking lotion, etc.)?
- Does this business anticipate a large number of walk-ins, or will the schedule be predictable far in advance?
- How does the scheduling process work, and who is responsible for it?
- How will the business attract new clients?
- How long is a session—does one hour actually mean 50 minutes?

There are no wrong answers to these questions, but it is important that employer and employee have the same standards. There should be reasonable boundaries that prioritize the health and longevity of the therapist and the well-being of clients. It is, unfortunately, far too common for large companies to only think of the bottom line, resulting in injury and disappointment.

Business Planning
Many massage therapists share the dream of opening a private practice. Therapists can legally work from home (if the space meets certain guidelines), or they can rent a room to host private clients. Many of these practices fail, due to improper planning. It is important to have a very specific plan before opening a business and brainstorm ways to make a business unique. How much capital is necessary to open a private practice? How much does one massage need to cost in order to meet revenue goals? What is the cheapest way to do laundry on a daily basis without sacrificing hygienic standards? No matter how talented a therapist is at massage, it is important to have a solid plan.

Strategic Planning
Strategic planning in the healthcare business has some unique facets. A private practice is built one client at a time. However, it is hard to build that practice without a space to host private clients. Being a business owner comes with much more freedom and much more responsibility than being an employee. Some practices succeed with just one therapist; others need to hire more employees to account for overflow. There are pros and cons to any decision a business owner makes, including legal business structure. Massage therapists who are looking to start their own practice should think ahead, consult professionals and experts, and work towards specific goals whenever possible.

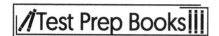

Office Management

Managing a medical office, such as those for massage therapists, comes with its own unique challenges. HIPAA, or the Health Insurance Portability and Accountability Act, strictly regulates recordkeeping procedures and requirements. For example, it is unacceptable to write SOAP notes in the body of an email sent to an employee, and written consent must be obtained from a client to share their medical information. In addition to the business of running an office—communicating with insurance companies, keeping client records, and so forth—clients expect certain fixtures in a medical office, such as tissues, cough drops, and filtered water. If possible, massage therapists should choose an office that is wheelchair accessible so no potential client is turned away. These seemingly small details send the message that the therapist cares deeply for clients and prioritizes their physical comfort, which enhances client satisfaction.

Appointment scheduling and client intake forms should be completed in the front office, if such a space is available at the office or spa. It is important to have a friendly and knowledgeable front desk staff to greet clients and make them feel welcome. HIPAA laws are not enforced in a non-medical, third-party carrier facility, however client confidentiality, even at the front desk, must always be respected and maintained.

Marketing

Marketing strategies depend on the scope of a therapist's practice and the business model. The following are some marketing tips for various kinds of business models:

Private Practice

The client base of a self-employed therapist is built slowly. The therapist's personal contacts will be their first clients, and news of the business will spread through recommendations from those clients. Every single relationship is important, and gaining one client will open doors to many more over time. It can be beneficial to offer referral bonuses to loyal customers—the industry standard is a half-hour massage for every referred friend who becomes a regular client. Online marketing can be done through social media, blogging, and online advertising. It is always best for the therapist to meet potential clients in person, if possible, so the client and therapist can assess compatibility. Some clinics offer community care events or healing circles where therapists, acupuncturists, and other healthcare providers can meet and connect with potential clients; these are excellent opportunities for small businesses to grow.

Medical Clinics

Marketing massage therapy in a hospital or chiropractic clinic has a unique set of challenges and opportunities. While these clients are seeking relief for specific pains and ailments, they are still in need of relaxation and respite from excessive stress, which could be exacerbating their medical conditions. A benefit for therapists working with clients in a medical facility is that, under certain circumstances, a client's medical insurance will cover at least part of a massage therapy session. This is often a deciding factor for whether a client in that environment wants a massage. Doctors or chiropractors who prescribe massage for patients as part of their treatment are a key part of marketing as referral sources for such clinics.

Spas and Hotels

Marketing massage therapy in a spa, hotel, resort, or other relaxed setting is straightforward because these sites attract clients with money to spend and an interest in pampering themselves. The therapist should approach each guest with consideration of their needs over all else, remembering that massage

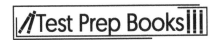
is not just in the healthcare industry, but falls within the service industry as well. Therapists should try to learn as much as possible about the client's needs and offer a service that seems well-suited to them.

Hiring/Interviewing

The hiring process for a massage therapist is unique. All interviews should include a practical component in which the therapist works on the interviewer or another staff member. Therapists are cautioned to be wary about interviewing for jobs that do not require practicals, as this indicates that the employer might not care about the skill sets of their employees. Practical interviews can sometimes be awkward; in no other profession is the interviewee expected to touch their potential employer's naked body within minutes of meeting for the first time. However, this awkwardness fades with practice, confidence, and time.

Documentation and Records

Client Records

It is important to keep records in accordance with HIPAA regulations, even though they do not legally apply outside of a medical facility that deals with insurance companies. Nonetheless, confidentiality is paramount; client records should never be shared with anyone unauthorized to view them. Typically, the only people authorized to view a client's health history are clients themselves, other therapists, and the client's medical team. In some cases, a client's legal guardian will also have access to this information. These records are important for a number of reasons:

- Client records help the therapist devise a treatment plan. If a client responds poorly to cryotherapy, for instance, the therapist should not prescribe ice packs to treat a newer injury.
- In case of any legal dispute, records protect the therapist. If a client suffers from severe, sudden-onset back pain after a massage, there's a chance the therapist will be legally implicated. The therapist's records are the only hard evidence that can be used to determine the facts in this kind of dispute.

Business Records

Accurate bookkeeping is important for taxes, insurance claims, and marketing and protects a business from financial confusion and scrutiny. This is especially important in an industry where tipping is commonplace; the therapist must record income both before and after tips. It can also be helpful to track demographic information about clients. A business that serves only new mothers will need to use different marketing and business tactics than one geared toward professional athletes. Finally, scheduling is a uniquely important aspect of this field. Double-booking clients or cancelling on them at the last minute can severely impact client retention rate. It is vital to be clear and communicative with everyone who walks through the door, and good recordkeeping practices allow the therapist to do just that.

Health Care and Business Terminology

- **Acupuncture:** An ancient style of Eastern medicine currently enjoying a resurgence in the West. Acupuncturists use needles placed at specific points in the body. Many acupuncturists also prescribe herbs and supplements. This modality can be used to treat a variety of physical and mental maladies.

109

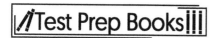

- **Alexander Technique:** A style of movement and body awareness developed by F.M. Alexander to keep the skeletal system in alignment during daily activities. Practitioners of this technique hold private and group sessions, teaching clients how to improve their posture with minimal physical touch.

- **Adjustment:** A chiropractic adjustment releases the gas that accumulates in joint capsules due to regular wear and tear, poor posture, and/or acute injury. Some people think of this process as "cracking" the back, although this term is not used by practitioners.

- **Alternative medicine:** A catch-all phrase used to describe medicine outside the typical doctor-patient relationship in the United States. Alternative medicine can refer to Eastern medicine of any kind, massage therapy, meditation, functional medicine, etc.

- **Aromatherapy:** The use of scents to serve a specific purpose. For example, lavender oil can be used to alleviate anxiety. Massage lotion can be infused with essential oils, or scents can be diffused throughout the treatment room.

- **Bodyworker:** A catch-all term for any healthcare provider who works directly with the client's body. Massage therapists, acupuncturists, physical therapists, and even estheticians might be referred to as bodyworkers. The term connotes a certain level of personal connection between the provider and client; it is not usually applied to doctors.

- **Chair massage:** Massage offered to a client seated in a special massage chair, often used as a business promotion. Massage chairs are highly portable, and clients are not required to disrobe; for that reason, these massages can be offered for shorter sessions (usually 10-15 minutes) in public settings.

- **Commission:** The percentage of revenue that a massage therapist is paid. If the therapist's commission is 50% and a client pays $100 for a massage, the LMT makes $50. This does not include tips. If an employer pays therapists based on commission, it is usually because they offer massages at different rates—one price for a sports massage, another price for a Swedish massage, etc. It is important for the therapist to carefully track these changing rates and their own daily sessions.

- **Complimentary massage:** A free massage. If the LMT is an independent contractor, they should not expect to be paid for this kind of work. Complimentary massages are useful promotional tools.

- **Contraindications:** Medical issues that preclude a client from receiving a service. For example, massage is contraindicated when a client has the flu.

- **Co-pay:** The amount of money an insured client is expected to pay for one office visit. For example, a clinic offers massages for both insured and uninsured clients. A self-pay massage is $100. One client's insurance will cover massages, but lists the co-pay as $10. The therapist would charge the client $10 on the day they perform the treatment and expect a further $90 from the insurance company after submitting a claim.

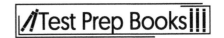

- **Craniosacral therapy:** A modality in which the massage therapist manipulates the cranium, spine, and sacrum. This style of massage is intended to improve the flow of cerebrospinal fluid through the body. It is viewed by some as energy work.

- **Cryotherapy:** The branch of hydrotherapy using cold temperatures. Ice and ice packs are applied to acute injuries to control inflammation and decrease pain.

- **Cupping:** A modality using cups applied to the skin to produce intense suction. This breaks up superficial fascial adhesions and causes the deeper muscles in the area to relax. Cupping is sometimes painful and usually causes dark bruising that heals over a few days.

- **Deductible:** A set amount of money that the client must pay before their insurance begins to cover the costs of care. The better the insurance plan, the lower the deductible. High deductibles can be a barrier to patients seeking the treatment they need.

- **Deep tissue massage:** Massage using consistently deep and specific pressure, reaching the deeper layers of muscle versus the superficial ones addressed during Swedish massage. Clients seeking deep tissue massage typically have a high pain tolerance (or think that they do).

- **Employee:** When a therapist works as an employee of a company rather than a contractor. Employees can either be paid by the hour or by commission, and the employer will deduct payroll and Social Security taxes. The tax burden is lower than for a contractor, but the take-home pay may decrease as a result. The main benefit of working as an employee is that the therapist may have a more regular schedule of steady clients.

- **Energy work:** Any modality that focuses on the supposed energy of the client or the supposed exchange of energy between client and provider. Some forms of energy work also include physical touch; some are purely meditative. Reiki is a common example of energy work.

- **Esalen:** A specific style of relaxation massage developed in California that uses a combination of techniques, but consists mainly of long strokes performed while the massage therapist is in a meditative state, which allows for intuitive responses to the needs of the client's body. Esalen requires many hours of training and is highly sought after by clients at upscale hotels and spas.

- **E-stim:** The gentle electric stimulation of specific muscles to cause deep relaxation after an injury. E-stim is not appropriate for all clients, but a doctor may prescribe it if a muscle is in severe spasm.

- **Face massage:** Commonly offered in spa and hotel settings, face massage can certainly be medical if intended to relieve sinus pressure, headaches, or similar symptoms. Most often, though, this is purely a relaxation technique.

- **Facials:** Not to be confused with face massage, facials use creams, ointments, and chemicals to improve the client's skin. They are usually provided by licensed estheticians.

- **Functional medicine:** A style of Western medicine that focuses on the patient's diet. Many people turn to functional medicine in response to gastrointestinal conditions such as Crohn's, IBS, and unexplained weight loss or gain.

111

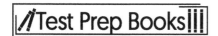

- **Gait analysis:** The study and analysis of a person's gait (the way they walk). It is possible to learn a great deal about a client's posture by looking at their movement patterns.

- **HIPAA:** An acronym for Health Insurance Portability and Accountability Act. HIPAA regulates many aspects of health care, but it is most notable for its impact on confidentiality. Every healthcare professional should be familiar with the many details of HIPAA. For instance, it is illegal to share any information about a client publicly, including their name and specific treatment plan. It is also illegal to email a client with treatment-specific information, unless that client actively requests that the therapist do so. The details of HIPAA are changing rapidly to keep up with evolving technology.

- **Holistic medicine:** A catch-all term used to describe medicine that considers the client's entire self during treatment. Acupuncture, for instance, uses the same techniques to treat physical and emotional health—as such, it is a holistic form of medicine. Putting a broken arm in a cast may be effective treatment, but it is not holistic.

- **Hot stone massage:** The application of smooth river stones, heated in a crock pot or hydrocollator, directly on the client during a massage. Hot stone massage requires special training and can also be a form of energy work.

- **Hours per week:** Not a complicated term, but a confusing concept. Therapists should only commit to the number of hours per week they can reasonably work without injuring themselves. Additionally, they should be aware of how many massages their employer expects to receive each day; being at work for 40 hours a week might not be difficult if the therapist only offers two hours of massage per day. Also, pay close attention to breaks. Having a consistent 15 minutes to recover between sessions can make or break a therapist's longevity.

- **Hydrocollator:** A machine that uses hot water to warm up heat packs. Most hydrocollators are electric and immerse the heat packs directly into the hot water, so they are wet to the touch. It is important to keep tongs and towels on hand to avoid being scalded.

- **Hydrotherapy:** Meaning "water therapy," it refers to the therapeutic use of temperature. Examples include applying an ice pack or a heating pad to the injured area.

- **Independent contractor:** It is common for therapists to work as independent contractors. Under this type of contract, the employer is not responsible for paying payroll or Social Security taxes. As a result, the therapist's take-home pay is higher. However, therapists are responsible for paying those taxes on a quarterly basis. Therapists will only be paid for time spent doing massages. Unfortunately, it is quite common for employers to require therapists to be present for an entire shift, even under these terms. It can be frustrating to spend an eight-hour day at work, only to be paid for two hours of work.

- **Insurance claim:** The statement a healthcare provider makes to an insurance company about a service performed. For example, a chiropractor might submit a claim that lists the number of adjustments, massages, and traction sessions that a client received. This is a step in the process of reimbursement.

- **Intake evaluation:** Each client's health status should be evaluated thoroughly before the first session with a new therapist and discussed briefly before every ensuing treatment. It is best for

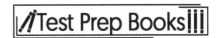

an intake evaluation to include a written component so the therapist can keep records of the client's medical history, prescriptions, and insurance information. The intake should also include a conversation so the therapist can get a more complete understanding of how that medical history impacts the client's daily health and mood.

- **Manual therapy:** In a clinical setting, such as a chiropractic clinic, a massage therapist's work will be billed to insurance as manual therapy. It is often measured in units of 10-15 minutes.

- **Myofascial release:** A style of bodywork focusing on the client's fascia, or connective tissue. MFR techniques are usually performed without lotion or oil. They represent a way to stretch muscles and tendons, break up adhesions, and eliminate scar tissue.

- **Out-of-pocket maximum:** The maximum amount of money an insurance plan will allow a patient to pay for care in a given year.

- **Palpation:** The use of touch to identify a specific muscle or anatomical structure. In a job interview at a chiropractic clinic, a therapist might be asked to palpate each of the erector spinae separately. It is rare but not unheard of for employers to test a therapist's palpation before hiring them.

- **Physical therapy:** The stretches and exercises prescribed by a doctor or physical therapist to aid a client's healing process. PT is sometimes performed in the clinic with the physical therapist on hand to guide the client. It can also be recommended that the patient perform certain activities on their own time.

- **Plumb line:** A string or wire attached to the ceiling of the room and weighted so it falls perfectly perpendicular to the ground. This is a valuable tool for postural analysis. Have the client stand beside or behind a plumb line to see whether their spine and other joints are out of alignment from their center of gravity.

- **Practical:** Shorthand for "practical interview," the portion of a job interview where the therapist performs a massage. It is common for the therapist to work on their potential employer.

- **PROM:** An acronym for pain-free range of motion, a term describing the maximum possible ROM of a joint before the client feels discomfort. Like ROM, it is a valuable assessment tool.

- **Re-exam:** An appointment with a doctor or bodyworker to discuss the client's progress. Chiropractors typically schedule a re-exam with each patient 2-4 weeks into their treatment plan.

- **Reflexology:** Massage applied to the feet. Reflexologists study the connection between certain areas of the foot and various internal organs and bodily systems. For instance, a reflexologist might apply pressure to the sole of the foot in order to relieve gastric distress.

- **Rehab:** In the field of bodywork, this usually refers to the rehabilitation of injured muscles. (In layman's terms, it is more often used to describe recovery from addiction.) Rehab specialists or physical therapists work with clients to stretch and strengthen muscles as part of the healing process.

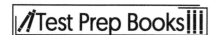
- **Reiki:** A form of energy work where the practitioner supposedly transfers energy from themselves to the client through their hands.

- **Report of findings:** A medical term often used in chiropractic settings. The ROF describes a doctor's opinion about the patient's diagnosis and recommended treatment plan. It is usually presented to the patient as a formal report during their second appointment.

- **ROM:** Range of motion of a particular joint measured in degrees. Measuring ROM is an easy way to track the effects of manual therapy.

- **Scalp massage:** Often used as a relaxation technique by therapists working in spas or hotels. It can also be a pointed, effective part of certain modalities, including craniosacral massage. Most clients have strong feelings about scalp massage in one way or another—it is best to ask before using it in a treatment.

- **Sharps:** Needles used in treatment. These can include acupuncture needles, hypodermic needles, and more. Sharps must be disposed of according to FDA regulations.

- **Shiatsu:** A Japanese massage modality that means "finger pressure." The therapist may apply pressure using their hands and feet, as well as stretches, along the traditional Chinese medicine meridian system.

- **SOAP notes:** A therapist working for a doctor may be required to take formal notes. Most often, they follow this format. SOAP is an acronym for Subjective observations, Objective observations, Assessment, and Plan.

- **Specialization:** Most established massage therapists specialize in one or more styles of bodywork. This is a great way to target a particular demographic, hone a specific skill, and build a private practice. A therapist might specialize in sports massage, prenatal, lymphatic drainage, or any number of modalities.

- **Sports massage:** Massage for athletes, often offered at gyms or sporting events. Massage can be helpful immediately before or after an event for athletes to maintain their bodies. Many people seek sports massage whether or not they are athletes; non-athletes usually use this term to refer to deep, vigorous, energizing bodywork.

- **Standard precautions:** A set of control practices set forth by the CDC to limit the spread of infection. Closely related to universal precautions, standard precautions include such common practices as frequent hand-washing and changing sheets between clients.

- **Tips** (or **gratuities**): Most practices allow massage therapists to accept tips from clients. It is customary for clients to tip 20% in spas and hotels. Tips are far more variable in medical settings; some clients don't tip at all, especially if their treatment is covered by insurance.

- **Traction:** Tractioning techniques elongate the joints, most often the spine. A chiropractor's office might have a traction table, for example. This machine is not unlike the massage chairs in a nail salon, except that it is much more clinical and specific. The client lies supine on the table, the doctor sets a timer, and a pin moves along the client's spine for a set amount of time

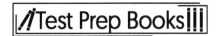

(usually 5-7 minutes), releasing the erector spinae. Traction can also refer to manual techniques employed during a massage to lengthen the torso or a limb.

- **Treatment plan:** The actions a medical provider takes to heal a client. The therapist should come up with a flexible plan that allows for the vagaries of life. A client with carpal tunnel syndrome might heal more quickly if they stop typing for a few weeks, but if they have a desk job, that is not feasible. If the therapist collaborates with the client to set realistic intentions, there's a better chance that healing will be fast and thorough.

- **Universal precautions:** A standardized set of rules in the healthcare industry to prevent the spread of infection. In a nutshell, universal precautions limit contact with bodily fluids.

Practice Test #1

1. What term describes a microorganism that causes a disease?
   a. Pathogen
   b. Virus
   c. Prion
   d. Vector

2. A person has inflammation of the synovial sheet of a connective tissue. What is the term for this condition?
   a. Emphysema
   b. Tuberculosis
   c. Tenosynovitis
   d. Peritonitis

3. Compression massage involves:
   a. Stretching the targeted muscle and then contracting against resistance
   b. Pressing into muscles with a steady tempo to engage the tissue
   c. Rubbing perpendicular to the grain of the muscle fibers
   d. Gentle massage of the muscles using kneading and gliding techniques

4. Varicose veins are:
   a. Shrunken veins that protrude from the skin
   b. Veins in the arms that appear bright red
   c. Swollen veins that are visible beneath the skin
   d. Veins that are surrounded by contusions or hematomas

5. What does the term myalgia refer to?
   a. Joint stiffness
   b. Chronic inflammation from uric acid crystals
   c. Inflammation that leads to fusion of spinal joints
   d. Muscle aches

6. In which location would voluntary striated muscle be present?
   a. Heart
   b. Intestinal walls
   c. Neck
   d. Stomach

7. Which is the common term for the medical condition, caused by repetitive arm motion, known as lateral epicondylitis?
   a. Tennis elbow
   b. UCL injury
   c. ACL injury
   d. Torn Achilles tendon

8. Which of the following describes the sutures of the skull?
   a. Amphiarthrosis
   b. Synarthrosis
   c. Diarthrosis
   d. Biarthrosis

9. When a massage therapist is working with a client, they completely control the movement of their client's joint while the client's muscles are completely relaxed. What type of range of motion is this considered for the client's joint?
   a. Active range of motion
   b. Fluid range of motion
   c. Resisted range of motion
   d. Passive range of motion

10. When the therapist uses pressure from their core through extended limbs to apply pressure to the client directly from the center of gravity, this is called:
   a. Distribution of force
   b. Lines of force
   c. Maximum possible pressure
   d. Bodily alignment

11. How does prenatal massage help expectant mothers deal with edema?
   a. It can help drain fluid from swollen tissues and joints.
   b. It relieves tension and tightness in the lumbar and hips.
   c. It stretches and compresses the entire body for stress relief.
   d. It provides heat to deep layers of the muscle.

12. A centripetal massage movement is directed towards which structure?
   a. Heart
   b. Neck
   c. Arm
   d. Leg

13. Which of the following is a concave structure that holds another bone in place to form a ball-and-socket joint?
   a. Epiphysis
   b. Acetabulum
   c. Ischium
   d. Ilium

14. Which movement of the thumb is perpendicular to the plane of thumbnail and parallel to the palm?
   a. Opposition
   b. Flexion
   c. Adduction
   d. Extension

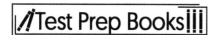

15. What does the positive rest position involve?
    a. Stretching the erector spinae from the iliac crest to the cervical vertebrae
    b. Standing with the back and arms flush against the wall
    c. Lying on the side while elevating the knee
    d. Lying on the back with knees raised on a pillow

16. Massage therapy strokes should always move in which direction?
    a. Distally, away from the heart
    b. From the front of the body toward the back
    c. From the top of the head down toward the toes
    d. Proximally, toward the heart

17. Muscle fibers are bound together into parallel structures known as what?
    a. Myofibrils
    b. Perimysium
    c. Sarcolemma
    d. Fasciculi

18. Which part of the trapezius muscle originates from a location on the occipital bone?
    a. Descending
    b. Middle
    c. Transverse
    d. Ascending

19. How should a client's private records be secured?
    a. All records should be printed and physically locked in a filing cabinet.
    b. All records should be electronic and should be password protected.
    c. Records should either be locked in a filing cabinet or password-protected on a computer.
    d. Records should be safeguarded and kept with the therapist at all times.

20. Which structure is an invagination of the plasma membrane in striated muscle that has several ion channels to allow excitation-contraction coupling?
    a. T-tubule
    b. Vesicle
    c. Acetylcholine
    d. Myofibril

21. What does the acronym PROM stand for?
    a. Pain-free range of motion
    b. Potential range of motion
    c. Pain-free range of movement
    d. Potential range of movement

118

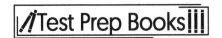

22. A person eats cake, which causes their blood sugar to increase. As a result, their pancreas releases insulin which lowers their blood sugar. What form of feedback mechanism is this an example of?
    a. Positive feedback
    b. Negative feedback
    c. Neutral feedback
    d. This is not an example of a feedback mechanism.

23. A patient has permanently tightened muscles and tendons that cause a joint to become stiff and lose much of its range of motion. What is this condition known as?
    a. Contracture
    b. Muscle cramp
    c. Fracture
    d. Tendonitis

24. Which condition is a result of damaged valves in the veins?
    a. Varicose vein
    b. Hemophilia
    c. Ulcer
    d. Aneurysm

25. The term "draping" refers to:
    a. Ensuring that window treatments effectively block windows and provide privacy for the client
    b. Covering a client with sheets for modesty and the comfort of the client
    c. Taking the time to be respectful and hang the client's clothing during the session
    d. Making sure that the massage table is clean and sterilized before each session

26. Which muscle is involved in a medial rotation of the arm?
    a. Pectoralis major
    b. Erector spinae
    c. Rhomboids
    d. Biceps brachii

27. What does the acronym ABMP stand for?
    a. Associated Bodywork and Massage Panel
    b. American Bodywork and Masseuse Providers
    c. Alliance of Bodywork and Massage Professionals
    d. Associated Bodywork and Massage Professionals

28. A massage therapist can demonstrate additional education and training by becoming board certified through which organization?
    a. ABMP
    b. AMTA
    c. NCBTMB
    d. COMTA

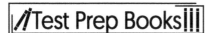

29. Which area of the body is affected by plantar fasciitis?
    a. Ankle
    b. Heel
    c. Palm
    d. Knee

30. How long is a typical chair massage?
    a. Five to ten minutes
    b. Ten to twenty minutes
    c. Thirty minutes
    d. Forty-five minutes

31. A person is diagnosed with a condition that results in vertebral arches not fusing into spinous processes. Which condition is this?
    a. Torticollis
    b. Kyphosis
    c. Scoliosis
    d. Spina bifida

32. A massage therapist develops personal, romantic feelings towards a client several months after the client began receiving therapy services. This is an example of a(n):
    a. HIPAA violation
    b. Dual relationship
    c. Transference
    d. Countertransference

33. What is the definition of anatomy?
    a. How the structure and systems of the body work together
    b. The location and physical structure of the parts of the body
    c. The composition of scar tissue versus healthy muscle
    d. The study of inflammation and the healing process

34. Bones are connected to one another by which structure?
    a. Tendon
    b. Cartilage
    c. Ligament
    d. Actin filament

35. How does access to a patient's health records help the massage therapist devise a treatment plan?
    a. The records can tell the therapist if the client has any treatment preferences.
    b. The records can assist the therapist in knowing whether certain therapy methods would be contraindicated.
    c. The therapist can determine if the patient is being treated by appropriate medical professionals.
    d. The therapist can assess the effectiveness of the procedures and prescriptions made by the client's doctors.

36. Pain that stems from a damaged internal organ is known as what?
    a. Chronic pain
    b. Visceral pain
    c. Somatic pain
    d. Acute pain

37. What is the first phase in the therapist-client relationship?
    a. Scheduling
    b. Intake
    c. Diagnosis
    d. Treatment plan

38. Why is it important for massage therapists to have a full understanding of both anatomy and physiology?
    a. To know when to refer a client to a doctor for additional care
    b. To know when a problem is physical or psychological in nature
    c. To understand how problems with the physical body and its systems can be affected by various techniques and treatment methods
    d. To determine when a client is suffering from inflammation rather than just muscle tension

39. Reflexology uses pressure points in what part of the body?
    a. The back
    b. The hands
    c. The feet
    d. It depends on which part of the body needs treatment

40. Which body system is most directly impacted by massage?
    a. Skeletal
    b. Vascular
    c. Digestive
    d. Neurological

41. What is the term for a condition involving systemic pain, fatigue, and muscle tenderness?
    a. Fibromyalgia
    b. Depression
    c. Anxiety
    d. Hypertonic tissue disease

42. Massage therapists must avoid contact with a client's bodily fluids to prevent the spread of bacteria and infectious diseases. Which of the following is NOT considered an infectious bodily fluid?
    a. Perspiration
    b. Mucus
    c. Saliva
    d. Vaginal secretions

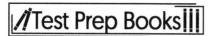

43. Which of the following most closely defines prone and supine?
    a. Prone means standing still, while supine means engaging in movement.
    b. Prone means engaging in movement, while supine means standing still.
    c. Prone means lying on the stomach, and supine means lying face up.
    d. Prone means lying face up, while supine means lying on the stomach.

44. Which of the following conditions is infectious?
    a. Ganglion cyst
    b. Atopic dermatitis
    c. Scabies
    d. Scleroderma

45. What does the deep friction technique called "clearing" involve?
    a. Reminding the brain of old injuries to stimulate nociceptors at the site
    b. A gradual increase of pain designed to overwhelm the Golgi tendon organs
    c. A quick jolt of pain designed to shut down the Golgi tendon organs
    d. Waking up the nervous system to increase the client's energy

46. The brachial plexus can be damaged when which muscle is massaged with too much pressure?
    a. Teres minor
    b. Frontalis
    c. Trapezius
    d. Scalenes

47. Which of the following is NOT a requirement for obtaining and maintaining a massage therapy license?
    a. Submitting an application to the licensing board
    b. Completing a course of education from an accredited school
    c. Passing the licensing exam
    d. Paying annual renewal fees

48. Which bone can be found in the neck?
    a. Hyoid
    b. Xiphoid process
    c. Ethmoid
    d. Patella

49. Which of the following terms best describes a gland?
    a. Control center
    b. Effector
    c. Stimulus
    d. Receptor

50. Reiki is a practice involving the movement of:
    a. Energy
    b. Blood flow
    c. Deep tissue
    d. Facial muscles

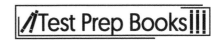

51. Due to decreased clot-dissolving abilities, pregnant massage patients are at higher risk for developing which issue?
    a. Aneurysm
    b. Cardiac arrest
    c. Deep vein thrombosis
    d. Hemophilia
    d. Methods of preparing and sanitizing a room for a session

52. What is the effect of dopamine on the body?
    a. It increases feelings of pleasure and motivation.
    b. It increases feelings of happiness and well-being.
    c. It increases the ability to bond with other humans.
    d. It increases the body's response to physical stress.

53. Which of these is NOT a benefit of massage for those struggling with substance addiction?
    a. An increase in dopamine
    b. Establishing reliable boundaries in relationships
    c. Having someone to talk to
    d. Chemical treatments for withdrawal

54. The shoulder and hip are examples of which classification of joint?
    a. Uniaxial
    b. Multiaxial
    c. Diaxial
    d. Biaxial

55. What are the meridians and the chi in shiatsu massage?
    a. The middle cross lines of the body and the movement of the massage pressure
    b. The vertical line down the middle of the body and the type of finger pressured used in the massage
    c. The specific pressure points targeted in the massage and the body's energy flow
    d. The body's energy pathways and the energy flow

56. What is the purpose of a hydrocollator?
    a. It dries a client's perspiration.
    b. It cools water for cryotherapy uses.
    c. It warms up heat packs.
    d. It cleans and sterilizes massage therapy equipment.

57. Which of the following terms describes the study of the nature and cause of diseases?
    a. Pathology
    b. Microbiology
    c. Virology
    d. Histology

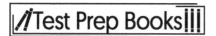

58. Which term refers to the use of cold therapy to control inflammation?
    a. Hypertonic
    b. PRICE
    c. Cryotherapy
    d. Edema

59. Forward head posture is most commonly seen in which group(s) of clients?
    a. Pregnant women and new mothers
    b. Students and office employees
    c. Elderly clients
    d. Scoliosis patients

60. What does the term "contraindications" mean?
    a. Treatments that should not be performed at the same time
    b. Unexpressed discomfort by the client
    c. Performing modalities that are counter to the client's pain tolerance
    d. Conditions or symptoms that are reasons a client should not receive a particular treatment

61. How can stress cause physical damage to the body?
    a. Increased levels of dopamine, serotonin, and oxytocin cause muscles to tighten and become painful.
    b. Emotional stress makes people sleep more, causing muscles to become stiff and sore.
    c. Increased levels of cortisol, epinephrine, and norepinephrine make muscles tight and painful.
    d. Stress at work causes people to need more time off, which causes more stress over finances and job security.

62. What is effleurage?
    a. A deep-tissue kneading technique
    b. A quick, percussive stroke
    c. Physical manipulation of a joint
    d. A gliding stroke that provides constant pressure

63. Which of the following is an example of an ethics violation?
    a. The therapist plays loud rock music that the client dislikes during an appointment.
    b. The therapist is ten minutes late to the appointment, but calls to let the client know and gives them a discount on the session.
    c. The client dislikes the therapist's loud pink hair color and complains to the manager.
    d. The client reports that the therapist was making crude jokes during the session and made fun of the client for complaining.

64. The amount of money an insured client must pay for a session is called a:
    a. Session rate
    b. Complimentary rate
    c. Commission
    d. Co-pay

65. What are the three planes of the body?
    a. Sagittal, mid-sagittal, and coronal
    b. Mid-sagittal, coronal, and transverse
    c. Sagittal, coronal, and transverse
    d. Mid-sagittal, mid-axial, and transverse

66. What is the purpose of professional liability insurance?
    a. It protects the client in the event of a mistake by the therapist.
    b. It protects the therapist against damages to the building, office space, and equipment.
    c. It protects the therapist against client injury and malpractice lawsuits.
    d. It protects the property owner in the event of a lawsuit against the property.

67. A therapist massages a clients' carotid sinus. How would the clients' body react to this action?
    a. Decrease in blood pressure
    b. Release of dopamine
    c. Increase in body temperature
    d. Activation of neck muscles

68. Which gait may indicate neurological problems?
    a. Antalgic
    b. Ataxic
    c. Anthrogenic
    d. Trendelenburg

69. The telencephalon matures into which structure?
    a. Cerebellum
    b. Cerebrum
    c. Ventricle
    d. Gyrus

70. What is ischemia?
    a. Fibrous connective tissue between muscles and organs
    b. A restriction in the blood supply
    c. A pebble-like texture underneath the skin
    d. The body's fight-or-flight response

71. Which is NOT an indication of client discomfort when conducting the passive range of motion exercises?
    a. Verbal expression
    b. Slow, deep breathing
    c. Facial expressions
    d. Tense or resistant tissue

72. Which muscle originates at the scapula?
    a. Pectoralis major
    b. Pectoralis minor
    c. Teres major
    d. Serratus anterior

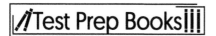

73. Gait analysis is the study of:
    a. The way a person moves from stand to sit and back to stand
    b. The way a person stands
    c. The way a person walks
    d. The way a person moves while adjusting their body position

74. Which is NOT considered a normal type of body movement?
    a. Supination
    b. Adduction
    c. Hyperflexion
    d. Extension

75. How can a massage therapist maintain professional boundaries with their clients?
    a. Avoid volunteering personal information and details.
    b. Avoid casual conversation during sessions; discuss only the client's physical health needs.
    c. If working from home, explain to clients that this is a personal living space, and it is not open to the public.
    d. Avoid returning any flirtatious behavior or sexual conversation except when pursuing a more personal relationship with the client.

76. What are the two branches of the autonomic nervous system?
    a. The sympathetic nervous system and the parasympathetic nervous system
    b. The sympathetic nervous system and the biosympathetic nervous system
    c. The parasympathetic nervous system and the neurosympathetic nervous system
    d. The biosympathetic nervous system and the neurosympathetic nervous system

77. What extra care might be required for a patient with high anxiety?
    a. More compressions, rocking, and soothing strokes prior to deeper massage techniques
    b. Deep breathing and steady, percussive massage techniques
    c. Additional stretches and periods of rest
    d. Extra time to analyze the client's posture and gait

78. The pyloric sphincter separates the stomach from which structure?
    a. Ileum
    b. Duodenum
    c. Esophagus
    d. Jejunum

79. A person has a respiratory disorder. As a result, the oxygen levels in their blood are reduced. What is this condition known as?
    a. Hypoxia
    b. Edema
    c. Anemia
    d. Oxytetracycline

80. What does psoas refer to?
   a. A muscle
   b. A massage technique
   c. An injury
   d. A type of gait

81. What is the best course of action should a therapist or client develop feelings outside of the professional relationship?
   a. Proceed with the professional relationship while exploring a more personal connection outside of the therapy sessions.
   b. Terminate the professional relationship and refer the client to another therapist.
   c. Discuss the situation and determine the best way forward together as a team.
   d. Ignore the feelings and work to maintain the professional relationship.

82. What is the typical cause of acute muscle pain?
   a. Physical defects
   b. Repetitive use
   c. Overuse
   d. Injury

83. Why should massage therapists avoid wearing perfumes or other strongly scented hygiene products?
   a. Wearing scented products could be seen as unprofessional.
   b. Perfumes and the like are generally against office policies.
   c. The licensing laws prohibit using scented hygiene products.
   d. Clients may be sensitive to smells and find the scents unpleasant.

84. What is the Alexander Technique?
   a. A style of treatment that uses needles placed at specific points on the body to treat pain
   b. A chiropractic technique used to release gas in the joints
   c. The use of various scents to serve specific purposes, such as alleviating anxiety
   d. A system that uses minimal touch while teaching clients how to maintain skeletal alignment during regular activities

85. Why is communication of utmost importance in massage therapy?
   a. Therapists must be able to present their information and requests to licensing agencies.
   b. Therapists must be able to communicate effectively with lawmakers regarding licensing issues.
   c. Therapists must be able to communicate clearly and effectively with clients, other therapists, and employers.
   d. Therapists must be able to clearly communicate their ideas in advertising and marketing campaigns.

86. Shoulder flexion and transverse adduction occurs due to which muscle working as a synergist to the pectoralis major?
   a. Anterior deltoid
   b. Innermost intercostals
   c. Psoas major
   d. Gluteus maximus

127

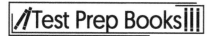

87. A steppage gait is due to a weakness in which muscles?
    a. Hip adductors
    b. Glutes
    c. Pelvic muscles
    d. Dorsiflexors

88. Why is communication important during the service phase of the therapist-client relationship?
    a. The therapist needs to assess the client's comfort level during the session.
    b. The therapist should engage the client in conversation to help the client feel at ease.
    c. The therapist should tell the client what they are doing during each step of the therapy session.
    d. The therapist should explain each modality during the session so the client understands what treatment methods are being employed.

89. What condition is Bruegger's relief position used to treat?
    a. Swayback
    b. Lordosis
    c. Kyphotic posture
    d. Bridges

90. What does HIPAA stand for?
    a. Health Insurance Portability and Accountability Act
    b. Health Information Privacy and Portability Act
    c. Health Information Patient Privacy Act
    d. Health Insurance Patient Privacy and Accountability

91. In which structure would one find oxygenated blood?
    a. Pulmonary vein
    b. Right atrium
    c. Inferior vena cava
    d. Right ventricle

92. What should a massage therapist do if they have a minor cut or a wound on their hands or fingers?
    a. Refer the client to another massage therapist.
    b. Clean their hands thoroughly using an antibacterial soap or sanitizer before and after the session.
    c. Wear a latex glove or finger cot to protect against infection.
    d. Cancel the appointment and reschedule when the wound heals.

93. Which organ is NOT found within the abdominal cavity?
    a. Thymus gland
    b. Ileum
    c. Spleen
    d. Gallbladder

94. What information is included under the activity section of the SOAP notes?
    a. The client's health concerns
    b. Tests and assessments of the client's posture, gait, and motion
    c. Anticipated plans for continuing care
    d. Performed procedures and treatment outcomes

95. Laws and regulations for massage therapy are set by:
    a. The federal government
    b. Each county
    c. The states
    d. Each city

96. Which of the following is an example of a dual relationship?
    a. The client is the co-worker of the therapist's sister.
    b. The client is the manager of the local bank.
    c. The client is a police officer in the therapist's neighborhood.
    d. The client is the therapist's roommate.

97. The interview process for new massage therapists usually includes a practical component, which is a way for the employer to assess the candidate's:
    a. Massage skills
    b. Knowledge of the laws and regulations regarding massage therapy
    c. Understanding of office procedures

98. What is a "covered entity" with regards to patient confidentiality?
    a. Any medical provider who charges money for a service
    b. Any medical provider who transmits medical information to third parties
    c. Any medical provider who is not bound by HIPAA
    d. Any medical provider who works with the public

99. What should a therapist do to add a new modality to their scope of practice?
    a. Read numerous articles and studies about the new modality.
    b. Complete thorough, accredited, and hands-on training in the new modality.
    c. Watch others perform the new treatment modality to fully understand its application.
    d. Discuss the new treatment modality with their office or practice manager.

100. A style of bodywork that focuses on connective tissue is called:
    a. Myofascial release
    b. Craniosacral therapy
    c. Facials
    d. Functional medicine

Answer Explanations #1

1. A: A pathogen is a bacterium that invades a body, causing infection. Choice *B*, virus, is incorrect because, while viruses can cause disease and in many cases are considered pathogens, they do not always cause diseases. Choice *C*, prion, is incorrect because it is a protein that causes other proteins to fold improperly. Choice *D*, vector, is incorrect because it is a living organism that transmits a form of pathogen.

2. C: Tenosynovitis is an inflammation of a tendon and the synovial sheath of that tendon. Choice *A*, emphysema, is incorrect because that describes a condition where the lungs are damaged by inhaling particulates, resulting in difficulty breathing. Choice *B*, tuberculosis, is incorrect because it is a bacterial infection of the lungs. Choice *D*, peritonitis, is incorrect because it refers to an inflammation of the peritoneum, a membrane that lines the inner abdominal wall.

3. B: Compression massage involves pressing into the muscles, either along or against the grain of the fibers, with a steady tempo. Choice *A* refers to muscle energy technique, which is commonly used with athletes. Choice *C* refers to cross-fiber frication, and Choice *D* refers to effleurage and petrissage techniques.

4. C: Varicose veins are swollen veins that are visible beneath the skin. Choice *A* is incorrect as the veins are not shrunken, though they can sometimes protrude from the skin. Choice *B* is incorrect, as varicose veins usually have a blue appearance. Choice *D* refers to bruising.

5. D: Myalgia is a term for muscle aches and pains, so Choice *D* is correct. Choice *A*, joint stiffness, is incorrect because myalgia refers to muscle aches. A common cause of joint stiffness is a condition known as arthritis. Choice *B*, chronic inflammation from uric acid crystals, is incorrect because that is a condition known as gout. Choice *C*, inflammation that leads to fusion of spinal joints, is incorrect because that is a condition known as ankylosing spondylitis.

6. C: The neck is the correct answer because it is controlled by voluntary skeletal muscles. Skeletal muscles are striated muscles that are not controlled by the somatic nervous system, meaning that they can be voluntarily activated. Striated muscles are muscles with thick and thin filaments known as sarcomeres, while smooth muscles have no sarcomeres. Choice *A*, heart, is incorrect because cardiac muscles in the heart are involuntary and controlled by the autonomic nervous system, even though they are also striated. Choices *B* and *D*, intestinal walls and stomach, are incorrect because they contain involuntary smooth muscles.

7. A: Tennis elbow is the common name for lateral epicondylitis. Tennis elbow is swelling or a tear in the tendons of the forearm that bend one's wrist away from the palm. Choice *B*, UCL injury, is incorrect because that effects the medial side of the elbow, whereas lateral epicondylitis effects the lateral side of the elbow. Choice *C*, ACL injury, is incorrect because the ACL (anterior cruciate ligament) is a part of the knee joint. Choice *D*, torn Achilles tendon, is incorrect because the Achilles tendon connects the calf muscle to the bone of the heel.

8. B: Synarthrosis is correct because it is an immovable and fixed joint. Skull sutures are fixed joints that do not move at all. Choice *A*, amphiarthrosis, is incorrect because it refers to a partially movable joint, such as the pubic symphysis. Choice *C*, diarthrosis, is incorrect because it refers to a joint that allows

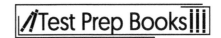

free movement, such as the elbow or shoulder. Choice *D*, biarthrosis, is incorrect because it is not a term for a joint.

9. D: Passive range of motion is the correct answer because this term refers to the motion of a massage therapist completely controlling a relaxed joint. This can be used to assess the complete mobility of a joint. Choice *A*, active range of motion, is incorrect because this is when a client uses their muscles to move a joint. Choice *B*, fluid range of motion, is incorrect because it is not a term used to describe a joint's range of motion. Choice *C*, resisted range of motion, is incorrect because this is when a client uses their muscles to show range of motion while a therapist applies resistance.

10. B: Lines of force refer to using pressure from the therapist's core through extended limbs to apply pressure to the client from the therapist's center of gravity. Choice *A*, distribution of force, refers to using correct hand positions to evenly distribute the force up the arm. Using proper lines of force allows for maximum possible pressure, Choice *C*, without injury to the therapist. Choice *D* is a made-up answer.

11. A: Edema refers to fluid retention and swelling in the extremities experienced by many pregnant women. Prenatal massage helps to drain this fluid from swollen tissues and joints. Prenatal massage can relieve tension and tightness in the lumbar and hips, but Choice *B* refers to sciatica, not edema. Choice *C* refers to Thai massage, and Choice *D* refers to hot stone massage, neither of which are specific to prenatal massage, so those choices are incorrect.

12. A: A centripetal massage movement is directed towards the heart, so Choice *A* is correct. All other choices—neck, arm, and leg—are incorrect because centripetal is defined as "towards the center." The neck, arms, and legs are away from the center of the body.

13. B: Acetabulum is the correct answer because it is the concave joint socket of the hip where the head of the femur attaches to make a ball-and-socket joint. Choice *A*, epiphysis, is incorrect because that is a round structure at the end of some bones, such as the femur. Choice *C*, ischium, is incorrect because it refers to a bone of the pelvis, although it does form a portion of the acetabulum. Choice *D*, ilium, is incorrect; it is also a pelvic bone that makes up part of the acetabulum.

14. B: Flexion is the correct answer because thumb flexion is a movement of the thumb on the frontal plane towards the palm. Choice *A*, opposition, is incorrect because thumb opposition movement is the movement of the thumb to meet the middle finger. Choice *C*, adduction is incorrect because thumb adduction is a movement on the sagittal plane. Choice *D*, extension, is incorrect because it is a movement on the frontal plane where the thumb moves away from the palm.

15. A: The positive rest position involves stretching the erector spinae by lying on the floor with the buttocks against the wall and the legs raised up the wall in a 90-degree position. Choice B refers to the beginning position for wall angels, while Choice C refers to the gluteus medius exercise. Choice D is incorrect, though this position can be helpful for clients who cannot lay comfortably flat on their backs.

16. D: To best improve circulation, massage strokes should always move proximally towards the heart. Choice A is the opposite of this, and Choices B and C are made-up answers.

17. D: Fasciculi, Choice *D*, refers to a group of muscle fibers bound together. Choice *A*, myofibrils, is incorrect because they are bundled proteins that contain the contractile portions of muscles. Choice *B*, perimysium, is incorrect because it is a connective tissue that surrounds and covers the fasciculus. Choice *C*, sarcolemma, is incorrect because it is a thin membrane that envelops each muscle fiber.

131

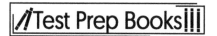

18. A: The descending part of the trapezius muscle, also known as the superior part, originates at the superior nuchal line and the external occipital protuberance of the occipital bone. Choice *B*, middle, is incorrect because no portion of the trapezius muscle is called the middle trapezius. Choice *C*, transverse, is incorrect because the transverse part of the trapezius muscle originates from the spinous processes of the cervical vertebrae and first three thoracic vertebrae. Choice *D*, ascending, is incorrect because this part of the muscle originates from the spinous processes of the rest of the thoracic vertebrae, T4 through T12.

19. C: Physical records and files should be kept in a locked filing cabinet, and electronic records should be password-protected. There is no need to make all records physical or electronic, as in Choices *A* and *B*, and the therapist physically holding onto all records, Choice *D*, is neither secure nor feasible.

20. A: T-tubule is the correct answer because it passes into muscle cells to spread an action potential. Choice *B*, vesicle, is incorrect because it is a small structure within a cell, made of a lipid bilayer enclosing fluid. Choice *C*, acetylcholine, is incorrect because it is a neurotransmitter at neuromuscular junctions. Choice *D*, myofibril, is incorrect because it is a bundle of muscle fibers.

21. A: PROM stands for pain-free range of motion, describing the maximum movement of a joint before the client feels pain. Choices *B*, *C*, and *D* are made-up answers.

22. B: Negative feedback is a regulatory process in which a stimulus triggers a reduction of the same stimulus. Choice *A*, positive feedback, is incorrect because that is a regulatory mechanism in which a stimulus results in an increase of the same stimulus. An example of a positive feedback mechanism is the process of contractions in childbirth. When contractions begin, they result in the release of oxytocin that triggers more contractions. Choice *C*, neutral feedback, is incorrect because that is not a regulatory feedback mechanism. Choice *D*, "This is not an example of a feedback mechanism," is incorrect because this scenario is an example of a negative feedback mechanism.

23. A: Contracture refers to a shortened and stiffened joint that occurs as a result of permanent tightening of muscles, tendons, and other tissues around a joint. Choice *B*, muscle cramp, is incorrect because that is a painful involuntary contraction of muscles that can occur due to strenuous use, dehydration, or lack of consistent use. Choice *C*, fracture, is incorrect because a fracture is a complete or partial break in a bone. Choice *D*, tendonitis, is incorrect because it refers to an inflammation of tendons that results in pain and a limited range of motion.

24. A: Varicose vein is the correct answer because it is an enlarged vein that occurs when valves within a vein are damaged. Choice *B*, hemophilia, is incorrect because that refers to a medical condition in which blood does not clot properly, making any bleeding wounds extremely dangerous. Choice *C*, ulcer, is incorrect because it is an open sore on an external or internal surface of the body. Choice *D*, aneurysm, is incorrect because that is when a blood vessel bulges from weakened vessel walls.

25. B: Draping refers to the use of sheets to cover a client for modesty and comfort. Sheets are also draped over the massage table for cleanliness and comfort. Choice *A* is important from a privacy standpoint, but this is not the definition of "draping." Choice *C* is not something the massage therapist should generally be concerned with. Choice *D* is vitally important, but is not the definition of "draping."

26. A: Pectoralis major is the correct answer because, along with the subscapularis, latissimus dorsi, teres major, and anterior fibers of deltoid, it is involved in the medial rotation of the arm. Choice *B*, erector spinae, is incorrect because the function of the erector spinae is to allow the vertebral column to

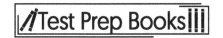

move. Choice *C*, rhomboids, is incorrect because these assist the movement of the scapula. Choice *D*, biceps brachii, is incorrect because it allows the flexion and supination of the forearm.

27. D: ABMP stands for Associated Bodywork and Massage Professionals, an industry organization that can help therapists obtain professional insurance. Choices *A*, *B*, and *C* are made-up answers and are therefore incorrect.

28. C: The National Certification Board for Therapeutic Massage and Bodywork is the governing body for board certification. Choices *A*, *B*, and *D* are other professional organizations providing insurance, continuing education opportunities, and support for massage therapists.

29. B: Heel is the correct answer because plantar fasciitis is an inflammation of the tissue that connects the heel to the toes. The pain from plantar fasciitis is located at the heel. Choice *A*, ankle, is incorrect because plantar fasciitis is only felt in the sole of the foot. Choices *C* and *D*, palm and knee, are incorrect because plantar refers to the sole of the foot, while the palm and knee are not structures of the foot.

30. B: A chair massage usually lasts about ten to twenty minutes and is a good modality for public places such as shopping malls and airports. Choices *A*, *C*, and *D*, then, are incorrect.

31. D: Spina bifida is the correct answer because it is a congenital defect of the spine that can cause paralysis of the lower limbs. Choice *A*, torticollis, is incorrect because it is a twist of the neck that results in the head being rotated and tilted at an angle. Choice *B*, kyphosis, is incorrect because it refers to an exaggerated bend in the spinal column. Choice *C*, scoliosis, is incorrect because it is an abnormal lateral curve in the spine.

32. D: Countertransference is when a therapist develops feelings for a client outside of the professional relationship. This is not a HIPAA violation, Choice *A*, which refers to sharing a client's medical records. Choice *B*, a dual relationship, is when a therapist and the client have a personal relationship prior to starting a professional therapy relationship. Choice *C*, transference, is when the client develops feelings for the therapist outside of the professional relationship.

33: B: Anatomy is defined as the location and physical structures of the body. Choice *A* is the definition of physiology. Choice *C* includes some anatomical information but is not the definition of the term, and Choice *D* refers to physiological information (though it is not the definition of physiology).

34. C: Ligament is correct because it is a dense elastic tissue that attaches bones to each other. Choice *A*, tendon, is incorrect because it is a connective tissue that is fibrous and attaches muscles to bone. Choice *B*, cartilage, is incorrect because it is a flexible connective tissue that functions as structural support and cushion throughout the body. Choice *D*, actin filament, is incorrect because it is a linear polymer that is important to muscle structure and function and to the formation of a cell's cytoskeleton.

35. B: The client's medical records can help a therapist determine if any particular treatment method would be contraindicated, such as using ice packs on a patient who does not handle cryotherapy well. Medical records do not usually include patient preferences, Choice *A*. In addition, while it is fine for a therapist to suggest medical attention for an undiagnosed issue or suggest the client seek a second opinion if the client is unhappy with their medical care, the therapist should not judge the medical qualifications of other professionals nor the treatments and prescriptions made by the client's medical team, as in Choices *C* and *D*.

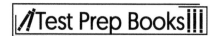

36. B: Visceral pain is the result of a damaged or malfunctioning internal organ, so Choice *B* is the correct answer. Choice *A*, chronic pain, is incorrect because that is pain that persists for an extended period of time. Choice *C*, somatic pain, is incorrect because that is pain that occurs due to activation of nociceptors in the muscles or on the surface of the body. Choice *D*, acute pain, is incorrect because that is sharp and suddenly occurring pain.

37. B: The first phase in the therapist-client relationship is intake. This is where the client and therapist communicate about the client's needs and concerns and establish a plan of action. While this first meeting may be scheduled, Choice *A* is incorrect. Therapists should not attempt to diagnose client issues, so Choice *C* is also incorrect. Finally, the therapist and client will devise a treatment plan together, but this is not the first phase of the relationship, so Choice *D* is incorrect.

38: C: It is important for massage therapists to have a full understanding of both anatomy and physiology because the body systems interact and work in conjunction with each other, and massage techniques and treatments depend on understanding how the body functions as a whole. While a therapist may need to sometimes refer a client to a physician for additional care, such as in Choice *A*, or may need an understanding of inflammation versus muscle tension, as in Choice *D*, these are not the full reason for studying both anatomy and physiology. Choice *B* is incorrect because the therapist should not make an assessment as to a client's psychological nature.

39. C: Reflexology involves specific pressure points in the feet that correspond to different parts of the body. Choices *A, B,* and *D* are all incorrect.

40. A: Massage most directly impacts the skeletal system. While other systems, such as those mentioned in Choices *B, C,* and *D*, might be positively affected, they are not the primary system massage therapy targets.

41. A: Fibromyalgia is a condition in which the patient suffers from systemic pain, near-constant fatigue, and muscle tenderness. Depression, Choice *B*, can be a potential cause for fibromyalgia, and anxiety, Choice *C*, can affect a client's well-being, but these are not the correct answer choices. Choice *D* is a made-up term. Hypertonic tissues have excessive muscle tone and can be tender or painful, but there is no specific disease for this condition.

42. A: Perspiration, or sweat, is not considered an infectious bodily fluid. Contact with the fluids in Choices *B, C,* and *D*, however, should be avoided.

43. C: Prone means lying on the stomach, while supine refers to lying face up. Choices *A* and *B* are incorrect, as prone and supine do not refer to motion but to position. Choice *D* is the opposite of the correct answer.

44. C: Scabies is an infectious condition in which skin becomes itchy from mites that burrow into the skin. Scabies can be passed from one person to another by physical contact or through contaminated items like bed sheets, clothing, or furniture. Choice *A*, ganglion cyst, is incorrect because that is a fluid-filled lump that typically occurs in the wrist and is not contagious. Choice *B*, atopic dermatitis, is incorrect because it refers to the non-infectious condition also known as eczema. It causes red, itchy skin and is common among children. Choice *D*, scleroderma, is incorrect because it is a type of rare non-contagious disease that results in the hardening and tightening of skin and some connective tissues.

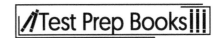

45. B: Clearing is a technique that gradually increases in pain in order to overwhelm the Golgi tendon organs and cause shutdown. Choice *C* is incorrect because the process is gradual, not quick. Choice *A* refers to trigger point therapy rather than clearing, and Choice *D* refers to the effect of using percussive strokes.

46. D: The scalene muscles are a group of muscles within the neck, above the brachial plexus. Choice *A*, teres minor, is incorrect because that is a narrow muscle in the shoulder. Choice *B*, frontalis, is incorrect because that refers to a superficial muscle in the forehead. Choice *C*, trapezius, is incorrect because that is a large muscle on the upper back.

47. A: The requirements for licensure include completing a course of education from an accredited school, passing the licensing exam, and paying the annual renewal fees, making Choices *B*, *C*, and *D* incorrect. A specific application submitted to the licensing board is not generally required, though state regulations may vary.

48. A: The hyoid is a U-shaped bone within the neck that provides support for the tongue and aids with swallowing and forming speech. Choice *B*, xiphoid process, is incorrect because it is located in the chest at the lower tip of the sternum. Choice *C*, ethmoid, is incorrect because that is one of the cranial bones forming the nasal cavity, nasal septum, and medial orbit wall. Choice *D*, patella, is incorrect because it refers to the floating bone within the knee.

49. B: An effector is an organ or structure that receives information from a control center so that it can produce a response. A gland receives information from the nervous system or endocrine system and responds by secreting something. For example, the sweat glands receive information from the hypothalamus and respond by producing sweat. Therefore, Choice *B* is correct. Choice *A*, control center, is incorrect because it receives information from a receptor, determines a response, and then sending a signal to an effector. An example of a control center would be the hypothalamus receiving information that the body is too cold from thermal receptors, then sending a signal to the muscles to begin shivering to produce heat. Choice *C*, stimulus, is incorrect because that would be something detected by a receptor, such as a bad smell that can be detected by olfactory receptors. Choice *D*, receptor, is incorrect because a receptor detects changes from normal conditions, then sends information to a control center. An example of a receptor is a nociceptor that detects pain to send a pain signal to the brain.

50. A: Reiki is a form of energy work that focuses on the movement of energy between the client and the practitioner. While it can include physical touch, it is often purely meditative. Choices *B*, *C*, and *D* all refer to more traditional means of massage therapy that stimulate circulation, apply pressure to deep tissue, and massage facial muscles, respectively.

51. C: Deep vein thrombosis is a condition, common in pregnant women, where clots form in deep veins. Choice *A*, aneurysm, is incorrect because it refers to a weakening of a blood vessel. Choice *B*, cardiac arrest, is incorrect because that happens when ones' heart stops unexpectedly. Choice *D*, hemophilia, is incorrect because it is a condition in which blood does not clot properly.

52. A: Dopamine production increases feelings of pleasure and motivation. Choice *B* is the effect of serotonin; Choice *C* is the effect of oxytocin. Choice *D* is incorrect because dopamine is not a response to stress, while a lack of dopamine could increase stress.

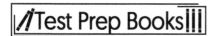

53. D: While massage therapy does increase dopamine as well as give patients a compassionate person to talk to who can help them re-establish reliable boundaries in relationships, the massage therapist does not prescribe chemical treatments for withdrawal. Choice *D*, therefore, is correct, while Choices *A, B,* and *C* are incorrect.

54. B: Multiaxial, also referred to as triaxial or polyaxial, is the correct answer because it is a type of joint that allows movement in three planes of motion. The hip and shoulder joints are considered multiaxial because they allow movement along three axes. Choice *A,* uniaxial, is incorrect because this type of joint only allows movement in a single plane. An example of a uniaxial joint is the elbow. Choice *C,* diaxial, is incorrect because it is not a term used to describe the motion capabilities of a joint. Choice *D,* biaxial, is incorrect because it is a joint that only allows movement along two axes. An example of a biaxial joint is the wrist.

55. D: In shiatsu massage, the meridians are the body's energy pathways, and the chi refers to the flow of energy throughout the body. Choices *A, B,* and *C* are all made-up answers and are therefore incorrect.

56. C: A hydrocollator is a machine that uses hot water to warm up heat packs. Choices *A, B,* and *D* are made-up answers.

57. A: Pathology is the study of the causes and effects of injuries and diseases. Choice *B,* microbiology, is incorrect because that is the study of microscopic organisms. Choice *C,* virology, is incorrect because that is the study of viruses and the diseases that arise from viruses. Choice *D,* histology, is incorrect because that is the study of biological tissues.

58. C: Cryotherapy refers to the use of cold therapy, such as cold packs, to reduce inflammation. Choice *B,* PRICE, refers to an acronym for remembering the different aspects of treating injuries (protection, rice, ice, compression, and elevation). Choice *A* refers to a muscle that is too tense or rigid while at rest, and Choice *D* refers to a condition involving a buildup of excess fluid in the body.

59. B: Forward head posture results from people who spend a great deal of time hunched over a computer or desk, so it is most commonly seen in students and office employees. Choices *A, C,* and *D* all have their own sets of common issues and therapies needed, but forward head posture is not the most common among these groups.

60. D: Contraindications are conditions or symptoms that would cause a client to react poorly to a particular treatment. Massage treatments and techniques should be carefully selected to make sure they do not exacerbate the client's existing health issues. Choices *A, B,* and *C* are made-up answers and are therefore incorrect.

61. C: Increased levels of cortisol, epinephrine, and norepinephrine that are generated by stress can make muscles tighten and become painful. Choice *A* is incorrect because dopamine, serotonin, and oxytocin improve the body's response to stress rather than causing more damage. Choice *B* is incorrect because stress usually results in a lack of restful sleep, not an increase in sleep. While stress at work can have the negative results in Choice *D,* those are not the physical results of stress.

62. D: Effleurage refers to a massage technique that provides a gliding stroke with constant pressure. Choice *A* refers to petrissage, Choice *B* refers to tapotement, and Choice *C* refers to joint mobilization, all of which are different types of massage techniques.

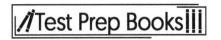

63. D: Making crude, rude, or otherwise offensive jokes during a session is an ethical violation that could result in the therapist being fired or even losing their license. Choices *A* and *B* are examples of service complaints. The practice manager may choose to address these issues with the therapist, but they would not be considered ethics violations. Choice *C* is a frivolous complaint made by the client and, unless the practice has a rule about hair color, would likely not result in any action against the therapist.

64. D: An insured client often has to cover a co-pay, which is the amount of money owed for the session that is not expected to be covered by insurance. Choice *A*, the session rate, is the amount of money charged by the massage therapist for the session. A complimentary massage, Choice *B*, is a free session that is often used as a promotion. Choice *C*, commission, refers to the percentage that the massage therapist makes when the revenue from the session is split between the therapist and the office or practice.

65. C: The three planes of the body are the sagittal (right and left), coronal (anterior and posterior), and transverse (upper and lower). The mid-sagittal line referenced in Choices *A*, *B*, and *D* is the midline of the body, and mid-axial is another name for the transverse plane.

66. C: Professional liability insurance protects the therapist against lawsuits due to client injuries or malpractice accusations. There are insurance policies available for the examples in Choices *A*, *B*, and *D*, but those situations are not covered by professional liability insurance.

67. A: Decrease in blood pressure is correct because baroreceptors reside within the carotid sinus. Pressure from massage will be detected by the baroreceptors, making the body attempt to lower the detected high pressure. Choice *B*, release of dopamine, is incorrect because dopamine's release is stimulated by pleasurable activities. Choice *C*, increase in body temperature, is incorrect because changes in blood pressure would most likely not affect body temperature. Choice *D*, activation of neck muscles, is incorrect because no structure within the carotid sinus triggers muscle contraction.

68. B: An ataxic gait involves staggering, weaving, or jerky movements, which are indications of a neurological problem. Choice *A* refers to a gait resulting from an injury. Choice *C* refers to the effects of osteoarthritis or rheumatoid arthritis, and Choice *D* refers to the effects of a weak or misfiring gluteus medius.

69. B: Telencephalon is the embryonic version of the cerebrum that eventually develops into an adult cerebrum. Choice *A*, cerebellum, is incorrect because that develops from the metencephalon. Choice *C*, ventricle, is incorrect because that is a type of heart chamber. Choice *D*, gyrus, is incorrect because that refers to a non-specific term for a ridge in the surface of the brain.

70. B: Ischemia refers to a restriction in the blood supply. Choice *A* refers to fascia. Choice *C* refers to how trigger points feel to the touch, and Choice *D* is governed by the sympathetic nervous system.

71. B: Clients who are experiencing discomfort will often indicate their discomfort through facial expressions, verbal indications, tight or resistant muscles and tissues, and rapid breathing. Choice *B* is the only option that does not indicate discomfort, making Choices *A*, *C*, and *D* incorrect.

72. C: Teres major is the correct answer because it originates from the scapula and inserts at the humerus. Choice *A*, pectoralis major, is incorrect because its origin is at the clavicle, sternum, and costal cartilage of the ribs. Choice *B*, pectoralis minor, is incorrect because its origin is at the anterior surfaces

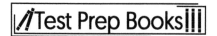

of ribs 3 to 5, and its insertion is at the scapula. Choice *D*, serratus anterior, is incorrect because its origin is at the ribs and its insertion is at the scapula.

73. C: Gait analysis refers to the study of the way a person walks. Choices *A, B,* and *D* are all made-up answers, though a massage therapist may be able to make some determinations as to the level and location of a client's pain based on how the clients stands and moves.

74. C: Hyperflexion is correct because, although it is a form of movement, is an excessive flexion of a limb beyond what is normal and could cause injury. Choice *A*, supination, is incorrect because it describes a rotation of the foot or the forearm toward standard anatomical position. Choice *B*, adduction, is incorrect because it refers to the movement of a limb toward the midline of the body. Choice *D*, extension, is incorrect because it is the movement that straightens joints.

75. A: There are several things a therapist can do to help maintain professional boundaries, including not discussing their own personal details or problems. Choices *B, C,* and *D* all include some incorrect information and/or are the opposite of what the therapist should do. In Choice *B*, it is fine to have casual conversation and for the client to share personal information, but the therapist should refrain from sharing their own personal information. If the therapist works from their home, as in Choice *C*, the workspace should be separate from their living space. Finally, if the client engages in flirtatious or sexually suggestive conversation, as in Choice *D*, the therapist should tell them that type of topic is unacceptable and that the session will be ended if it continues. The therapist should never engage in a personal relationship with a client.

76. A: The two branches of the autonomic nervous system are the sympathetic and the parasympathetic nervous systems. "Biosympathetic" and "neurosympathetic" are made-up terms, making Choices *B, C,* and *D* incorrect.

77. A: Clients who are exhibiting high levels of anxiety may require additional compressions, rocking, and soothing strokes to help them relax prior to deeper work. Choices *B, C,* and *D* are incorrect, though some of them can be used with clients, depending on their particular needs.

78. B: The pyloric sphincter separates the stomach from the duodenum, the first portion of the small intestines, so Choice *B* is the correct answer. Choice *A*, ileum, is incorrect because it is the last part of the small intestine and is separated from the cecum by the ileocecal valve. Choice *C*, esophagus, is incorrect because it is separated from the stomach by the lower esophageal sphincter. Choice *D*, jejunum, is incorrect because that term refers to the section of the small intestine between the duodenum and ileum.

79. A: Hypoxia is the medical term for oxygen levels in the blood being too low. Choice *B*, edema, is incorrect because it refers to swelling caused by fluid buildup in the body tissues. Choice *C*, anemia, is incorrect because that occurs when one's body does not produce enough healthy erythrocytes (red blood cells). Choice *D*, oxytetracycline, is incorrect because it is a type of antibiotic that kills a wide variety of microorganisms.

80. A: The psoas is the muscle that runs from the lower vertebrae to the anterior pelvis, making Choices *B, C,* and *D* incorrect.

81. B: If either the therapist or the client develops feelings for the other, the best course of action is to terminate the professional relationship and refer the client to another therapist. While a more personal

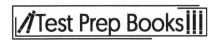

connection can be explored, as in Choice A, it should be done after the termination of the professional relationship. Communication is important, as in Choice C, but the therapist must be professional first and should make the decision to end the professional relationship. Choice D, trying to ignore the feelings, can cause tremendous problems and is the wrong path forward.

82. D: The most typical cause of acute muscle pain is from injury. While overuse and repetitive use, such as in Choices B and C, can cause acute muscle pain, they are not the most common cause. Choice A is not a cause of acute muscle pain and is incorrect.

83. D: Massage therapists should avoid wearing perfumes or other scented hygiene products because clients may be sensitive to smells and/or find the scent unpleasant. Offices and practices may establish rules about personal hygiene, as in Choice B, but the basis for rules like these stems from the comfort of the clients. While wearing or using scented products is not necessarily unprofessional nor against licensing laws, Choices A and C, those products are best avoided to prevent any issues.

84. D: The Alexander Technique is a style of movement and body awareness meant to help clients maintain proper skeletal alignment during daily activities. Choice A refers to acupuncture. Choice B refers to chiropractic adjustment, and Choice C is aromatherapy.

85. C: Therapists primarily communicate with clients, other therapists, and their employers on a regular and ongoing basis, making communication in these relationships of utmost importance. Choices A, B, and D may represent other areas of communication that could arise from time to time, but these are not usual or typically ongoing situations.

86. A: The anterior deltoid works as a synergist with the pectoralis major, allowing shoulder flexion and transverse adduction, making Choice A the correct answer. Choice B, innermost intercostals, is incorrect because these are deep muscles between the ribs that work as synergists for the movements of the internal intercostals. Choice C, psoas major, is incorrect because it does not work along with the pectoralis major for any movements. Choice D, gluteus maximus, is incorrect because it is takes part in many movements of the legs, whereas the pectoralis major is located on the thorax of the body.

87. D: A steppage gait results from weakness in the dorsiflexors, the muscles in the front of the shin. Weakness in the hip adductors, Choice A, can cause a scissors gait, while weakness in the glutes, Choice B, results in a lurching gait. Choice C is a made-up answer.

88. A: The therapist should check in with the client during the session to gauge their comfort with factors like the amount of pressure and temperature. Choices C and D are incorrect, as this level of discussion should be addressed before the session, not during it. Choice B is incorrect, as casual conversation is not recommended during a session.

89. C: Bruegger's relief position involves pressing the chin towards the chest to stretch the neck while rolling the shoulders back, a good treatment option for clients with kyphotic posture. Choice A is a common name for lordosis, Choice B, in which the client's pelvis is tilted. Choice D refers to a treatment for lordosis.

90: A: HIPAA stands for the Health Insurance Portability and Accountability Act, referring to the 1996 patient privacy law. Choices B, C, and D are made-up answers.

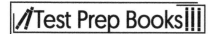

91. A: The pulmonary vein is the vessel that returns freshly oxygenated blood from the lungs back to the heart so that it can be pumped throughout the body. Choice *B*, right atrium, is incorrect because it is the chamber of the heart that receives deoxygenated blood from the vena cava. Choice *C*, inferior vena cava, is incorrect because it is a large vein that delivers deoxygenated blood to the heart. Choice *D*, right ventricle, is incorrect because it receives deoxygenated blood from the right atrium to pump to the lungs.

92. C: A therapist who has a cut or wound on their hand or finger should wear a latex glove or finger cot to prevent infection. There is usually no need to refer the client to someone else or to cancel the appointment, Choices *A* and *D*, unless the wound is severe enough to prevent the therapist from working at all. It is always a good idea to clean hands before and after a session, as in Choice *B*, but this is not specific to dealing with injuries.

93. A: Thymus gland is the correct answer because it is located in the thoracic cavity behind the sternum. Choice *B*, ileum, is incorrect because it is the final portion of the small intestine within the abdominal cavity. Choice *C*, spleen, is incorrect because it is located in the upper left portion of the abdominal cavity near the stomach. Choice *D*, gallbladder, is incorrect because it is located in the abdominal cavity, behind the liver.

94. D: The activity section of the SOAP notes includes the procedures performed by the therapist and the treatment outcomes, so Choice *D* is correct. Choice *A* refers to the subjective section of SOAP, while Choice *B* refers to the objective section and Choice *C* refers to the plan section.

95. C: Each state sets the laws and regulations for massage therapy. Choices *A, B,* and *D* are incorrect.

96. D: A dual relationship refers to situations in which the therapist is not only the client's therapist but is also their relative, friend, or business associate. In other words, there is some type of existing relationship in addition to the therapist-client relationship. Choices *A, B,* and *C* are not examples of dual relationships, unless the therapist is also friends with these people.

97. A: The practical component of an interview allows the employer to assess the candidate's massage skills and techniques. This is usually accomplished by having the potential employee perform a massage on the interviewer or another staff member. While the candidate may be asked about Choices *B, C,* and/or *D* during the interview, they are not part of the practical component.

98. B: Any medical provider who transmits medical information to third parties, such as insurance companies, is considered a "covered entity." Choices *A* and *D*, then, are incorrect. Choice *C* is incorrect due to the wording. A medical provider who IS bound by HIPAA is a "covered entity." Choice *C* says those who are NOT bound by HIPAA, which is incorrect.

99. B: To add a new treatment modality to their scope of practice, the therapist should undergo thorough, accredited, and hands-on training. While it is never a bad idea to read up on the new methods or to watch or discuss the method with others, Choices *A, C,* and *D* are insufficient preparation to offer a new treatment modality.

100. A: Myofascial release focuses on the fascia, or connective tissue, using stretching to break up adhesions and eliminate scar tissue. Craniosacral therapy, Choice *B*, focuses on the manipulation of the cranium, spine, and sacrum to improve the flow of cerebrospinal fluid. Choice *C*, facials, focus on

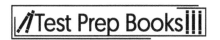

improving a client's skin and are usually provided by estheticians. Functional medicine, Choice *D*, is a style of medicine that focuses on a patient's diet.

Practice Test #2

1. Which of the following is NOT a purpose of the intake process?
   a. It keeps the therapist up to date regarding a client's health conditions.
   b. It demonstrates the therapist's commitment to the client's well-being.
   c. It sets up the treatment plan for the session.
   d. It allows time for the therapist and client to share small talk and personal discussions.

2. Massage therapy rules, mandates, and regulations are established by:
   a. Federal licensing boards
   b. The state health department
   c. The Federal Department of Health and Wellness
   d. State licensing boards

3. Which of the following can be an example of a saddle joint?
   a. Carpometacarpal joint
   b. Metacarpophalangeal joint
   c. Metatarsophalangeal joint
   d. Tarsometatarsal joint

4. What action is mediated by the triceps brachii muscle?
   a. Forearm extension
   b. Leg extension
   c. Forearm flexion
   d. Leg flexion

5. What is NOT a symptom of scoliosis?
   a. Muscle imbalance
   b. A slow, shuffling gait
   c. A weakening of the muscles on one side of the spine
   d. A curvature of the spine

6. Which of the following is NOT a consideration when starting a new practice?
   a. How much to pay licensed therapists compared to non-licensed therapists
   b. How many hours the therapists will work
   c. Who will manage the office, order supplies, and handle scheduling
   d. How the business will attract new clients

7. Which type of massage stroke involves using a kneading technique in deep-tissue work?
   a. Petrissage
   b. Effleurage
   c. Tapotement
   d. Stroking

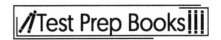

8. Which of the following is NOT one of the cerebral meninges?
   a. Arachnoid mater
   b. Dura mater
   c. Pia mater
   d. Subarachnoid mater

9. How often should the massage table and equipment be sanitized?
   a. At the start of each workday
   b. At the end of the workday
   c. Twice per week
   d. After each session

10. What are adhesions?
    a. Areas of excessive muscle tone due to tension in the spindle fibers
    b. The fibrous connective tissues between muscles and organs
    c. Bands of muscle fibers that stick together and form knots
    d. Pebble-like textures beneath the skin

11. Protecting a client's personal and medical information is a key aspect of what primary code of ethics?
    a. Transparency
    b. Professional courtesy
    c. Medical rights
    d. Confidentiality

12. Which muscle is necessary to flex the forearm at the elbow?
    a. Biceps brachii
    b. Brachioradialis
    c. Brachialis
    d. Supinator

13. What does the general/specific/general massage protocol involve?
    a. Using softer, gentle massage techniques before working towards deeper, more intense therapy, and then going back to more gentle massage
    b. Massaging the whole body or an entire area of the body before moving towards a certain issue or trouble area, and then moving back to the whole body or area
    c. Working on a body part from the section closer to the torso before moving to the areas farther away from the torso and then back
    d. Stretching the muscles both before and after any type of deep tissue massage therapies

14. Massage of varicose veins is usually contraindicated due to what possible complication?
    a. Pitted edema
    b. Embolism
    c. Infection
    d. Bruising

143

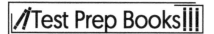

15. Which of the following is a term for a prediction of the outcome of a disease?
    a. Diagnosis
    b. Symptom
    c. Hypothesis
    d. Prognosis

16. Myosin binds with which structure to allow a sarcomere to contract?
    a. Actin
    b. Troponin
    c. Tropomyosin
    d. Myofibrils

17. A hemiplegic gait is the result of
    a. Long periods of immobilization
    b. Paralysis on one side of the body
    c. Weakness in the dorsiflexors
    d. Spasms in the psoas

18. Which plane divides the body into right and left halves?
    a. Coronal Plane
    b. Frontal plane
    c. Midsagittal plane
    d. Transverse plane

19. Which bone is NOT a portion of the axial skeleton?
    a. Pelvis
    b. Skull
    c. Rib
    d. Sacrum

20. What is the difference between pain and stress?
    a. Stress is trauma that occurs either physically or emotionally, and pain is the body's response to that trauma.
    b. Pain is the body's reaction to outside stimulus, while stress is the body's response to internal factors.
    c. Stress is an external response to emotional situations, while pain is the physical response.
    d. Pain is the body's alert system that something is damaged or injured, while stress is strain or tension that can be caused by physical or emotional triggers.

21. Which of the following is an example of the location of a gliding joint?
    a. Elbow
    b. Wrist
    c. Shoulder
    d. Skull

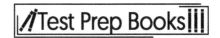
22. A person has small sacs protruding from their colon that become infected. What is this condition known as?
    a. Anaphylaxis
    b. Interstitial cystitis
    c. Gastroenteritis
    d. Diverticulitis

23. A person has completed all of the required education and has passed the licensing exam. Is this person able to legally practice massage therapy?
    a. Yes, they are fully educated and trained.
    b. Yes, they can practice while they await receipt of their license.
    c. No, they have not submitted an application for licensing.
    d. No, they have not provided the licensing agency with evidence of insurance.

24. Which is NOT a cancer of the skin?
    a. Basal cell carcinoma
    b. Squamous cell carcinoma
    c. Myeloma
    d. Melanoma

25. Which is an example of a condyloid joint?
    a. Elbow joint
    b. Wrist joint
    c. Intercarpal joint
    d. Thumb joint

26. Which of the following is a condition that someone could develop as a result of wearing a full leg cast for an extended amount of time?
    a. Leg fracture
    b. Varicose veins
    c. Sarcopenia
    d. Shingles

27. What does AMTA stand for?
    a. Association of Massage Therapists of America
    b. American Massage Therapists Association
    c. American Massage Therapy Association
    d. American Massage Therapists' Association

28. Which of the following is NOT a psychological benefit of touch?
    a. Increase in cortisol, epinephrine, and norepinephrine
    b. Release of serotonin, oxytocin, and dopamine
    c. Aids in forming attachments
    d. Helps generate feelings of compassion and respect

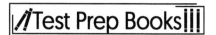

29. Which muscle is an antagonist of the subscapularis?
    a. External oblique
    b. Latissimus dorsi
    c. Teres minor
    d. Teres major

30. Wearing gloves while working with a minor cut or wound on the hands is beneficial in preventing the spread of bacteria and infection, but it also creates what negative issue?
    a. Gloves can lessen the ability to accurately feel the muscles while providing therapy.
    b. Gloves can give the impression that the client is somehow unclean and the therapist does not want to touch them.
    c. Gloves can become sticky or dirty during the session.
    d. Gloves can deteriorate and tear during the session.

31. All of the following are benefits of communication in the workplace EXCEPT:
    a. Clearly conveying a client's needs to each therapist who may work with that client
    b. Mentoring therapists who are new to the practice or new to massage therapy in general
    c. Enhancing employee relationships through casual chats and conversations
    d. Maintaining a well-run, transparent practice for employees

32. A massage therapist's client says they have a medical condition that results in repetitive twisting movements from involuntary muscle contractions. Which disorder or disease does this individual most likely have?
    a. Hypertension
    b. Dystonia
    c. Lupus
    d. Hepatitis

33. What is the technical term for a frozen shoulder?
    a. Adhesive capsulitis
    b. Tenosynovitis
    c. Hernia
    d. Lordosis

34. Sensory organs that provide information to the brain about muscle fiber, tendon tension, and joint angle positions are called:
    a. Spinal nerves
    b. Meninges
    c. Action potentials
    d. Proprioceptors

35. Lymphatic drainage massage can be helpful in clients who are suffering from
    a. Edema
    b. Hematomas
    c. Varicose veins
    d. Contusions

146

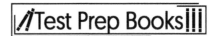

36. A client has osteoporosis. A massage therapist should avoid applying heavy pressure to which region?
    a. Thoracic cage
    b. Abdomen
    c. Thighs
    d. Upper arms

37. Strokes such as petrissage, tapotement, and effleurage are used primarily for what purpose?
    a. To increase circulation
    b. To release tight muscles
    c. To properly align the body
    d. To reduce stress in the body

38. Which of the following is the primary component of connective tissue?
    a. Hyaline
    b. Collagen
    c. Osteophyte
    d. Sarcomeres

39. Massage can help the body process and eliminate waste by increasing the flow of
    a. Oxygen
    b. Lymph
    c. Nutrients
    d. Blood

40. What is entrainment?
    a. The feeling the practitioner has of being in tune with the client
    b. The pathways that energy takes through the body
    c. The flow of energy through the body
    d. The "breath of life" used in craniosacral therapy

41. A muscle is not very flexible and has fascicles that attach obliquely to its tendon. Which muscle best fits this description?
    a. Psoas major
    b. Pectoralis major
    c. Biceps brachii
    d. Deltoid

42. Which of the following is NOT a factor to be considered in establishing and understanding scope of practice?
    a. Client preferences
    b. State laws and regulations
    c. Rules established by the practice
    d. Town ordinances

147

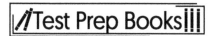

43. Which condition effects the gastrointestinal tract?
    a. Crohn's disease
    b. Tuberculosis
    c. Lou Gehrig's disease
    d. Glomerulonephritis

44. What is the appropriate temperature for the stones in hot stone massage?
    a. 100 to 120 degrees
    b. 120 to 150 degrees
    c. 150 to 180 degrees
    d. 180 to 200 degrees

45. The triceps brachii is an antagonist to which muscle?
    a. Pronation teres
    b. Teres major
    c. Deltoid
    d. Biceps brachii

46. What should a massage therapist do if they suspect that a client has an undiagnosed condition or medical issue?
    a. Ask the client probing questions to help ascertain if there really is a problem.
    b. Apply their anatomical and clinical knowledge to make a diagnosis of the problem.
    c. Nothing; it is against regulations to bring up any medical issues not part of the current treatment plan.
    d. Mention the possible concern to the client and suggest they speak with their doctor.

47. Which plane divides the body into upper and lower halves?
    a. Frontal plane
    b. Coronal plane
    c. Sagittal plane
    d. Transverse plane

48. Who is responsible for paying payroll and Social Security taxes for an independent contractor?
    a. The employer
    b. The contractor
    c. The IRS
    d. No one; independent contractors do not pay taxes

49. What is the purpose of using heat therapy during massage?
    a. Heat relieves inflammation to treat pain and swelling.
    b. Heat stimulates inflammation to relive tight or locked muscles.
    c. Heat is used with PRICE to treat acute pain, such as from an injury.
    d. Heat controls inflammation to prevent the body from further damaging itself.

50. Where is the cubital vein located?
    a. Elbow
    b. Knee
    c. Abdomen
    d. Lungs

51. Where should the massage therapist usually focus their gaze during a session?
    a. On the area of the body they are massaging
    b. On the client's face to assess if there is any visual display of discomfort
    c. Straight ahead, keeping the head and neck in proper alignment
    d. Wherever is most comfortable for the therapist and client

52. What is the definition of physiology?
    a. How the structure and systems of the body work together
    b. The location and physical structure of the parts of the body
    c. How oxygen moves through the lungs
    d. How inflammation affects scar tissue

53. The force required by a heart to pump blood out of the heart chambers is known as what?
    a. Blood pressure
    b. Atherosclerosis
    c. Systole
    d. Hypertension

54. The sole of a patient's foot is moved away from the median plane. What form of movement is this an example of?
    a. Inversion
    b. Pronation
    c. Eversion
    d. Supination

55. A dowager's hump often results from
    a. A forward head posture
    b. Tightness in the hip adductors
    c. Bruegger's relief position
    d. Lordosis

56. An injury to the foot, knee, ankle, or pelvis can result in which type of gait?
    a. Ataxic
    b. Antalgic
    c. Arthrogenic
    d. Lurching

57. Why should massage therapists avoid wearing fingernail polish?
    a. Nail polish can harbor bacteria.
    b. Wearing nail polish can be unattractive.
    c. Nail polish looks unprofessional.
    d. Wearing nail polish is against the professional code of conduct.

149

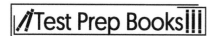

58. What course of action should be taken if the therapist makes an unwanted sexual advance towards a client?
    a. The therapist should be dismissed from the practice.
    b. The client should be dismissed from the practice for provoking the therapist.
    c. Another therapist in the practice should take over the client's care.
    d. The manager of the practice should take over the client's care.

59. A client has a condition where the myelin sheaths of many central nervous system nerve cells are damaged. What is the client's condition?
    a. Multiple sclerosis
    b. Parkinson's disease
    c. Dementia
    d. Alzheimer's disease

60. Trendelenburg gait can be detected by Trendelenburg's sign, which is
    a. Rigidity of the hip on the affected side
    b. A twisting of the hip on the affected side
    c. A dropping of the hip on the affected side
    d. A raising of the hip on the affected side

61. What does SOAP stand for?
    a. Service, Objective, Assignment, and Plan
    b. Subjective, Objective, Assessment, and Plan
    c. Subjective, Occupation, Assessment, and Procedure
    d. Source, Objective, Alignment, and Policies

62. Which of the following increases feelings of happiness and well-being?
    a. Oxytocin
    b. Dopamine
    c. Cortisol
    d. Serotonin

63. Transference is defined as:
    a. When a client develops feelings towards a therapist outside of a professional relationship
    b. When a therapist develops feelings towards a client outside of a professional relationship
    c. When a client begins working for the massage therapy practice
    d. When a therapist begins working for a new practice and brings their clients with them

64. A bacterial infection causes painful muscle contractions and eventually makes a person's neck and jaw muscles lock up. Which is most likely the reason for this condition?
    a. Malaria
    b. Psoriasis
    c. Tetanus
    d. Tuberculosis

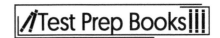

65. Tightness in the hip adductors, resulting in a scissors gait, is often seen in clients with which condition?
    a. Osteoarthritis
    b. Diabetes
    c. Parkinson's
    d. Cerebral palsy

66. Craniosacral therapy works with rhythms of the body known as the primary respiratory system to regulate the flow of:
    a. Blood
    b. Oxygen
    c. Cerebrospinal fluid
    d. Energy

67. What is a plumb line?
    a. A weighted string or wire attached to the ceiling and used to assess posture
    b. A line drawn on one wall of the therapy room and used to designate the center of the room
    c. A line drawn on the floor of the therapy room and used to assess a client's gait
    d. A line used to determine if the massage table is placed on a level surface

68. Which hormone is produced in higher amounts during pregnancy and can cause an increased risk for blood clots?
    a. Luteinizing hormone
    b. Aldosterone
    c. Estrogen
    d. Follicle stimulating hormone

69. An exercise involving standing with the back and arms against the wall and bringing the elbows in towards the body is called
    a. Pectoral muscle pinpoint
    b. Vertical rhomboid stretch
    c. Positive rest position
    d. Wall angels

70. Which function of the body is controlled by the parasympathetic nervous system?
    a. Involuntary functions such as respiration and circulation
    b. The fight-or-flight response
    c. The rest and digest functions
    d. Emotional responses

71. Which type of therapy involves placing needles at specific points in the body?
    a. Acupuncture
    b. Reflexology
    c. Cryotherapy
    d. Cupping

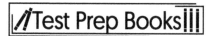

72. What does SOAP stand for?
    a. Strategies, objectives, achievements, proposals
    b. Strategies, objectives, assessment, plan
    c. Subjective, objective, assessment, plan
    d. Subject, orthopedics, analysis, procedures

73. Do HIPAA regulations apply to massage therapists?
    a. Yes, if they transmit medical information to third-party carriers such as insurance companies.
    b. Yes, all medical service providers are bound by HIPAA regulations.
    c. Yes, but only if they provide certain types of massage therapy techniques.
    d. No, massage therapists are not covered entities with regards to HIPAA.

74. Which massage modality centers around the movement of the body's energy flow?
    a. Swedish massage
    b. Reflexology
    c. Thai yoga massage
    d. Shiatsu

75. Which of the following is an example of a service complaint made by a client?
    a. The therapist did not address the client's lower back pain, even though the client expressly asked for care in that particular area.
    b. The therapist was ten minutes late for the appointment but ended the appointment on time, cutting the client's massage time short.
    c. The client complained that the therapist was telling inappropriate jokes and using crude humor during the session.
    d. A client complained that the therapist had to reschedule an appointment. The therapist gave the client three days' notice and offered the client a discount on the rescheduled appointment.

76. What term describes a circular movement of a limb that involves flexion, extension, adduction & abduction?
    a. Rotation
    b. Retraction
    c. Circumduction
    d. Protraction

77. How is connective tissue affected by aging?
    a. It becomes discolored.
    b. It is infected easily by pathogens.
    c. It renews itself.
    d. It becomes less pliable.

78. Who is typically authorized to view a client's medical records?
    a. The client, the massage therapist, and the client's immediate family
    b. The client, the client's spouse or immediate family, and the client's doctors
    c. The client and the client's legal guardian
    d. The client, the massage therapist, and the client's medical team

79. Which of the following is NOT part of a massage/bodywork session?
   a. Dietary evaluation
   b. Visual assessment
   c. Palpation assessment
   d. Clinical reasoning

80. Which cellular structure uses the metabolites from glycolysis to produce chemical energy?
   a. Mitochondria
   b. Sarcomere
   c. Cytoplasm
   d. Myocytes

81. The inguinal triangle is considered an endangerment site due to the presence of what structure?
   a. Pelvic bone
   b. Femoral nerve
   c. Aortic arch
   d. Hippocampus

82. Why is therapist-client communication important during the intake process?
   a. The therapist needs to explain to the client what services are offered by the practice.
   b. The client needs to feel comfortable enough to fully disclose their medical issues, concerns, and questions.
   c. The client must understand the laws and regulations governing their treatment options.
   d. The therapist needs to convince the client that their practice is the best place to receive treatment.

83. In addition to client privacy, what else is regulated by HIPAA?
   a. Office management policies, such as supply orders and employee work hours
   b. Which types of massage therapies are approved for the public
   c. Appropriate marketing strategies
   d. Record-keeping procedures and requirements

84. Which body system transports erythrocytes to supply cells with nutrients and oxygen?
   a. Respiratory
   b. Lymphatic
   c. Circulatory
   d. Integumentary

85. The two phases of the gait, when the foot is making contact with the ground and when the foot and leg are in the air, respectively, are called
   a. Stance and swing
   b. Swing and stance
   c. Lowered and elevated
   d. Elevated and lowered

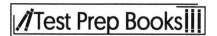

86. A massage therapist working on a client who is also their best friend is an example of a(n):
    a. Ethics violation
    b. Dual relationship
    c. Transference
    d. Countertransference

87. Oncology massage is directed at what primary benefit to the client?
    a. Promoting the movement of fluids to prevent edema
    b. Targeting specific areas of the body through pressure points in the feet
    c. Stretching the entire body for better range of motion
    d. Relieving the stress and anxiety of other medications and treatments

88. Which nerve runs from the lower back through the back of the thigh and down the lateral shins?
    a. Femoral nerve
    b. Lateral plantar nerve
    c. Sciatic nerve
    d. Peroneal nerve

89. Which phase of muscle contraction occurs when calcium ions, ATP, ADP, or ATPase are no longer available?
    a. Latent period
    b. Relaxation phase
    c. Excitation-contraction coupling phase
    d. ATP hydrolysis phase

90. What term refers to the region of the shoulder?
    a. Axillary
    b. Brachial
    c. Carpal
    d. Acromial

91. What can a massage therapist do when a client is unable to adequately explain a particular sensation or the exact location of pain during a session?
    a. Work around the general area, providing therapy to the entire region.
    b. Ask the client relevant questions to help pinpoint the location or issue.
    c. Read over the client's file to see if their doctor has provided more detailed information.
    d. Ask another therapist for their professional opinion on the problem and the best way to proceed.

92. Deep tissue massage may be contraindicated for all of the following EXCEPT:
    a. Recent injuries
    b. Diabetes
    c. Pregnancy
    d. Unregulated high blood pressure

93. Proprioception refers to:
    a. The body's sense of limb position and orientation in space
    b. The function of the nerves extending from each side of the spinal column
    c. The damage to the protective coverings of the central nervous system
    d. The lack of electrochemical signals from the neurons

94. What is E-stim?
    a. A type of relaxation massage often offered at upscale hotels and spas
    b. The application of smooth, heated stones directly onto the client's body
    c. An electric stimulation used to cause deep relaxation of the muscles
    d. The therapeutic use of temperature such as heating pads or ice packs

95. A set of control practices set forth by the CDC that limits the spread of infection is called:
    a. Cleanliness practices
    b. Common procedures
    c. Standard precautions
    d. Standard practices

96. What is NOT an aspect of the therapeutic relationship between a therapist and a client?
    a. Providing therapeutic services with compassion and patience
    b. Understanding the vulnerability of massage clients
    c. Diagnosing new or changing medical conditions
    d Staying in tune with the client's physical and emotional needs

97. Which of the following is considered a local contraindication?
    a. Varicose veins
    b. Neuritis
    c. Diabetes
    d. Cancer

98. How does environment impact the principle of stress reduction during a massage therapy session?
    a. A bright, clean, sterile environment promotes professional cleanliness.
    b. Bright lights and loud music promote a sense of fun and enjoyment.
    c. A well-appointed office setting demonstrates professionalism in the practice.
    d. Soft lighting and relaxing music promote relaxation.

99. Which of the following structures is NOT a portion of the alimentary canal?
    a. Kidney
    b. Mouth
    c. Rectum
    d. Pharynx

100. The alveoli are involved in which process?
    a. Gas exchange
    b. Blood filtration
    c. Fluid transport
    d. Antibody production

Answer Explanations #2

1. D: Therapists should avoid sharing personal details and too much casual conversation with clients in order to better maintain the professional relationship. Choices *A, B,* and *C,* however, list the benefits to conducting a thorough intake with each new client.

2. D: Massage therapy rules, mandates, and regulations are established by the licensing boards in each state. Choices *A, B,* and *C* are incorrect.

3. A: Carpometacarpal joint is the correct answer because the carpometacarpal joint of the thumb is a saddle joint. The only saddle joints of the body are found at the thumbs and the heels. Choice *B,* metacarpophalangeal joint, is incorrect because it is a multiaxial condyloid joint. Choice *C,* metatarsophalangeal joint, is incorrect because it is a type of ellipsoid synovial joint. Choice *D,* tarsometatarsal joint, is incorrect because the tarsometatarsal joints are examples of plane joints.

4. A: Forearm extension is the correct answer because the triceps brachii is located on the dorsal side of the upper arm and is responsible for extending the forearm. Choice *B,* leg extension, is incorrect because the quadriceps femoris is responsible for leg extensions. Choice *C,* forearm flexion, is incorrect because forearm flexion uses the biceps brachii muscle. Choice *D,* leg flexion, is incorrect because that is facilitated by the hamstring group of muscles.

5. B: A slow, shuffling gait can be a means of compensating for unsteadiness and is often seen in Parkinson's patients, not patients with scoliosis. Scoliosis is a mild to severe curvature of the spine, Choice *D,* that causes muscle imbalance, Choice *A,* and weakening of the muscles on one side of the spine or the other, Choice *C.*

6. A: A successful massage therapy business will never employ non-licensed therapists. Doing so could result in the loss of the business license and cause serious legal jeopardy. Choices *B, C,* and *D,* however, should all be considered to give the business the best chance of success.

7. A: Petrissage comes from the French word for "to knead" and involves using a kneading technique to focus on a particular muscle or knot. Choices *B, C,* and *D* all refer to other types of massage strokes.

8. D: Subarachnoid mater is the correct answer because it is not one of the cerebral meninges nor a name for a real structure in human anatomy. There is a region within the skull known as the subarachnoid space, but there is no subarachnoid mater. Choices *A, B,* and *C* are incorrect because they are the three cerebral meninges. The meninges are barriers that protect the brain and vessels within the skull. The dura mater is the outermost layer, the arachnoid mater is in the middle, and the pia mater is the innermost layer.

9. D: The massage table and equipment should be sanitized after each session to ensure that they remain clean and ready for each client. While a practice may have policies about sanitizing at the beginning or end of each workday or doing some type of deep clean periodically, Choices *A, B,* and *C,* those would be in addition to sanitizing after each session.

10. C: Adhesions are bands of muscle fibers that stick together and form knots. Choice *A* refers to hypertonic tissue. Choice *B,* the connective tissue between muscles and organs, is fascia, and Choice *D* describes trigger points.

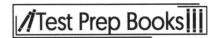

11. D: One of the primary aspects of a therapist's code of ethics is confidentiality with regards to a client's personal and medical information. Choices A, B, and C are made-up answers.

12. B: The brachioradialis is responsible for flexing the forearm at the elbow. It is a superficial muscle located at the lateral forearm. Choice A, biceps brachii, is incorrect because it flexes the elbow joint and supinates the hand and forearm. Choice C, brachialis, is incorrect because it only flexes the elbow. Choice D, supinator, is incorrect because it supinates the hand and laterally rotates the forearm.

13. B: The general/specific/general massage protocol involves massaging the whole body (or an entire area of the body, such as the whole back) before moving to focus on a particular problem area. Finish the massage by working back to the general techniques. Choice A is incorrect, as it describes the superficial/deep/superficial protocol. Choice C describes the proximal/distal/proximal protocol, and Choice D refers to simple stretching, which should be included with any treatment.

14. B: Massage of varicose veins poses the risk of embolism, the release of a potentially fatal blood clot. Pitted edema, Choice A, may indicate a cardiovascular or kidney condition, while any areas of infection or bruising, Choices C and D, should be avoided during any type of massage therapy.

15. D: Prognosis is a prediction of the outcome of a diagnosed disease. Choice A, diagnosis, is incorrect because that is the term for an identification of a disease, issue, or illness in a patient. Choice B, symptom, is incorrect because it refers to is the physical or mental result of a disease or other issue. Symptoms are signs of existence of an issue. Choice C, hypothesis, is incorrect because it is a proposed explanation for an event based on available evidence.

16. A: Actin is the correct answer because it binds to myosin heads to allow muscle contractions. Choice B, troponin, is incorrect because it is a protein along an actin filament that binds calcium ions. Choice C, tropomyosin, is incorrect because it is a protein on an actin filament that regulates muscle contraction and relaxation. Choice D, myofibrils, is incorrect because it is a functional unit of a muscle cell that performs muscle contractions.

17. B: A hemiplegic gait is the result of paralysis on one side of the body. It is most commonly seen in patients who have suffered a stroke. Choice A, Long periods of immobilization, such as in patients recovering from surgery, can cause muscle contracture and make walking difficult. Choice C, weakness in the dorsiflexors, results in a steppage gait, while spasms in the psoas, Choice D, cause a psoatic limp gait.

18. C: Midsagittal plane, also known as median plane, is the correct answer because it divides the body into equivalent right and left sides through the middle of the body. Choice A, coronal plane, is incorrect because that is a vertical plane through the body that separates it into dorsal and ventral halves, not right and left halves. Choice B, frontal plane, is incorrect because it is synonymous to a coronal plane. Choice D, transverse plane, is incorrect because it divides the body into superior and inferior parts.

19. A: Pelvis is the correct answer because the pelvis is a part of the appendicular skeleton. The axial skeleton is composed of the bones that make up the central axis of the body. The remaining bones are known as the appendicular skeleton and are the bones that attach to the axial skeleton. Choice B, skull, is incorrect because it aligns with the central axis of the body. Choice C, rib, is incorrect because it is at the center of the body, protecting vital organs. Choice D, sacrum, is incorrect because it is at the base of the spinal column and therefore a part of the axial skeleton.

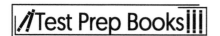

20. D: Pain is the body's way of telling us that something is wrong, like an alarm going off in the body. Stress is tension or strain that is the body's response to physical or emotional triggers. Choice *A* is incorrect because stress is not necessarily trauma, and pain is not always the body's response to stress. Choice *B* is incorrect because pain is not always only due to outside stimulus, and stress is not always a response to internal factors. Stress can be caused by external factors, such as a stressful job, and pain can be triggered by external injuries. Stress is often an internal response, rather than an external response, making Choice *C* incorrect.

21. B: Wrist is the correct answer because gliding joints exist in the wrist, ankle, and spine. Gliding joints, also known as planar joints, exist to allow bones to slide past each other in any direction. Choice *A*, elbow, is incorrect because the elbow is a hinged type of synovial joint. Choice *C*, shoulder, is incorrect because the shoulder is a ball-and-socket joint. Choice *D*, skull, is incorrect because the joints in the skull are immovable joints known as sutures.

22. D: Diverticulitis is an infection of small pouches that form in the intestines. Choice *A*, anaphylaxis, is incorrect because it is a severe allergic reaction that causes the body to release chemicals that make an individual go into shock. Choice *B*, interstitial cystitis, is incorrect because it is a condition that causes chronic bladder pressure and pain. Choice *C*, gastroenteritis, is incorrect because it is a stomach condition that is better known as a stomach flu.

23. C: To legally act as a massage therapist, one must not only complete all of the required education and training and pass the licensing exam, but must also submit an application to the licensing board, along with any required fees, and receive a valid license. This means Choices *A* and *B* are incorrect. While some states have certain insurance requirements, Choice *D*, that information is not usually required in order to obtain a license.

24. C: Myeloma is the correct answer because it is a cancer of plasma cells in the blood. Choice *A*, basal cell carcinoma, is incorrect because it is a skin cancer that develops in areas that are exposed to sunlight. Choice *B*, squamous cell carcinoma, is incorrect because it is the second most common form of skin cancer that causes abnormally accelerated squamous cell growth. Choice *D*, melanoma, is incorrect because it is a dangerous skin cancer that occurs when melanocytes become cancerous.

25. B: Wrist joint is the correct answer because it is a condyloid joint. This joint is a modified ball-and-socket movement and allows for the movement of the fingers. Choice *A*, elbow joint, is incorrect because it is a hinge joint. Choice *C*, intercarpal joint, is incorrect because it is a plane, or gliding, joint. Choice *D*, thumb joint, is incorrect because it is a saddle joint, which is another type of synovial joint.

26. C: Sarcopenia is the correct answer because it is a decreased muscle mass due to lack of activity. Casts prevent movement to allow bones to heal, which also prevent muscles from being used and results in lost muscle mass. Choice *A*, leg fracture, is incorrect because the purpose of a cast is to allow fractures to heal. Casts do not cause a bone to break. Choice *B*, varicose veins, is incorrect because they are enlarged and twisted veins that occur when high blood pressure weakens the walls of blood vessels. Choice *D*, shingles, is incorrect because it is a reactivation of the chickenpox virus that results in painful rashes.

27. C: The AMTA is the American Massage Therapy Association. Choices *A*, *B*, and *D* are made-up answers.

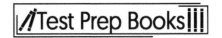

28. A: The increase in cortisol, epinephrine, and norepinephrine causes the muscles to become tight and painful, which is not a benefit of touch. There are many psychological benefits of touch, including the release of serotonin, oxytocin, and dopamine. This promotes feelings of happiness and increases feelings of compassion and respect, which can help people form stronger attachments to others, making Choices *B, C,* and *D* incorrect.

29. C: Teres minor is an antagonist of the subscapularis. Along with the infraspinatus, the teres minor relaxes when the subscapularis contracts and vice versa. Choice *A,* external oblique, is incorrect because the antagonists of the oblique muscles are the trunk extensor muscles, such as the erector spinae. Choice *B,* latissimus dorsi, is incorrect because its antagonist muscles are the deltoid and trapezius. Choice *D,* teres major, is incorrect because its antagonists are the anterior deltoid, middle deltoid, middle trapezius, and pectoralis minor.

30. B: Wearing gloves, while helpful in protecting a cut or wound on the therapist's hands, can give the impression that the therapist thinks the client is unclean and/or does not want to physically touch them. Wearing medically approved latex gloves will not detract from the therapist's ability to conduct an appropriate therapy session, Choice *A,* and if they become sticky, dirty, or tear during the session, as in Choices *C* and *D,* they can easily be replaced with a fresh pair.

31. C: While it is nice for employees to be friendly with one another and perhaps even develop relationships outside of the workplace, this is not an important consideration in workplace communication. Choices *A, B,* and *D* all demonstrate areas where communication is important in the workplace.

32. B: Dystonia is the correct answer because it is characterized by repetitive slow twisting movements as a result of involuntary muscle contractions. Choice *A,* hypertension, is incorrect because it refers to chronic high blood pressure. Choice *C,* lupus, is incorrect because lupus is an inflammatory disease where ones' immune system attacks their own tissues. Choice *D,* hepatitis, is incorrect because it is an inflammation of the liver.

33. A: Adhesive capsulitis is the term for a frozen shoulder, which causes stiffness and pain in the shoulder. Choice *B,* tenosynovitis, is incorrect because it refers to an inflammation of a tendon and its sheath. Choice *C,* hernia, is incorrect because that is a condition in which an organ pushes through a muscle or tissue. Choice *D,* lordosis, is incorrect because it is an inward curve of the lumbar portion of the spine.

34. D: Proprioceptors are sensory organs that provide information to the brain about muscle fiber, tendon tension, and joint angle positions. These organs include muscle spindles, Golgi tendon organs, and joint capsules. Choices *A, B,* and *C* refer to other parts of the nervous system. Spinal nerves extend from each side of the spinal column. Meninges are the central nervous system's protective coverings. Action potentials are electrochemical signals created by the neurons.

35. A: Edema is swelling that is caused by fluid retention. Lymphatic drainage massage can help release this fluid and thus reduce the swelling. Hematomas and contusions, Choices *B* and *D,* refer to bruising, and varicose veins, Choice *C,* are swollen veins that are visible beneath the skin.

36. A: Thoracic cage is the correct answer because osteoporosis can weaken bones, making pressure on thinner bones, like the ribs, particularly hazardous. Choice *B,* abdomen, is incorrect because there are no

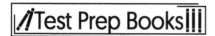

superficial and thinner bones within the abdomen. Choices *C* and *D*, thighs and upper arms, are incorrect because they contain the sturdier bones, the femur and humerus.

37. B: Effleurage, tapotement, and petrissage are strokes typically used in stretching and releasing tight muscles. Increasing circulation, Choice *A*, is one of the primary benefits of massage, and many strokes work towards that end, primarily in techniques such as Swedish and Thai yoga massage, but the strokes mentioned in the question are primarily used to ease the tension in tight muscles rather than focusing specifically on circulation. Massage does not generally work to align the body, Choice *C*, and while it can help to reduce a client's stress overall, Choice *D*, this is not usually achieved through specific techniques.

38. B: Collagen, Choice *B*, is the most abundant structural protein in connective tissue. Choice *A*, hyaline, is incorrect because that is a type of cartilage that provides support to joints and various other surfaces in the body. Choice *C*, osteophyte, is incorrect because an osteophyte is a protruding growth from a bone. Choice *D*, sarcomeres, is incorrect because these are a portion of striated muscles.

39. B: Massage can increase the flow of lymph, which helps aid in processing and eliminating waste. Massage does help to increase the flow of blood, which in turn increases oxygen and nutrients throughout the body, but those are not specific to waste, making Choices *A*, *C*, and *D* incorrect.

40. A: Entrainment refers to the practitioner's feeling of being in tune with the client during craniosacral therapy. While Choice *D* is also a craniosacral concept, it is not the definition of entrainment. Choices *B* and *C* refer to shiatsu massage concepts of the movement of energy (chi) through pathways in the body (meridians).

41. D: Deltoid is the correct answer because it is a pennate muscle. Pennate muscles are stronger, less flexible, and have fascicles that attach obliquely to its tendon. Choices *A* and *C*, psoas major and biceps brachii, are incorrect because they are examples of a fusiform muscle. Choice *B*, pectoralis major, is incorrect because it is an example of a convergent muscle.

42. A: The therapist needs to be aware of state laws and regulations as well as any specific town ordinances and the rules of the practice when understanding their scope of practice. Choices *B*, *C*, and *D* should be considered. While important for the therapist-client relationship and in determining a treatment plan, client preferences, Choice *A*, are not a part of establishing scope of practice.

43. A: Crohn's disease is the correct answer because it is an inflammation of a portion of the gastrointestinal tract. Choice *B*, tuberculosis, is incorrect because tuberculosis is an infectious disease caused by bacterial infection. Choice *C*, Lou Gehrig's disease, is incorrect because that is a nervous system disease. Choice *D*, glomerulonephritis, is incorrect because it is an inflammation and damage of the glomerulus in the kidney.

44. B: The stones for hot stone massage should be heated to a temperature between 120 and 150 degrees, making Choices *A*, *C*, and *D* incorrect.

45. D: Biceps brachii is an antagonist to triceps brachii. Antagonists relax and lengthen when their opposite muscle is flexed. Choice *A*, pronator teres, is incorrect because it is an antagonist to the supinator muscle. Choice *B*, teres major, is incorrect because it is an antagonist to various muscles such as the deltoids, middle trapezius, and pectoralis minor. Choice *C*, deltoid, is incorrect because it is not specific enough, as there are three separate deltoid muscle heads: the anterior, lateral, and posterior deltoids.

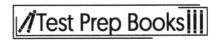

46. D: If the therapist suspects the client may have an undiagnosed medical condition or issue, they should mention their concern to the client and suggest the client make an appointment with their doctor. Choices *A* and *B* are incorrect, as the therapist should never try to diagnose an issue, even if they think they know what the problem might be. Choice *C* is also incorrect. While the therapist should not try to diagnose a problem, they should not ignore it either, particularly if the issue could be serious.

47. D: The transverse plane, also known as the horizontal, axial, or mid-axial plane, divides the body into upper and lower halves. The coronal plane, also known as the frontal plane, in Choices *A* and *B* divides the body into anterior and posterior, while the sagittal plane in Choice *C* divides the body into right and left.

48. B: An independent contractor is responsible for paying their own taxes. An employer pays taxes on behalf of their employees, as in Choice *A*. The IRS does not pay contractors' taxes for them, so Choice *C* is incorrect. Choice *D* is a common misconception. Independent contractors are just as responsible for paying taxes as any other working person.

49. B: Heat therapy is used to stimulate inflammation, which can help to relieve tight or locked muscles. Choices *A*, *C*, and *D* all refer to the use of cold therapies rather than heat.

50. A: Elbow is the correct answer because the cubital vein is located in the cubital fossa of the elbow. The cubital vein is a common location for needle insertion when drawing blood. Choice *B*, knee, is incorrect because the most prominent vein of the knee is the popliteal vein. Choice *C*, abdomen, is incorrect because the primary vein through the abdomen is the inferior vena cava. Choice *D*, lungs, is incorrect because the vein that delivers blood to the lungs is the pulmonary vein.

51. C: The therapist should focus their gaze straight ahead, keeping their head and neck in proper alignment in order to avoid any unnecessary strain on the head or neck. Occasionally the therapist will need to look at the area they are massaging, Choice *A*, but those are rare and specific instances. While the client may make some facial expressions during the session, staring at their face, Choice *B*, would only make both parties uncomfortable. While comfort is important, Choice *D* is incorrect because, while it may be comfortable to hang one's head or look around the room, this could result in strain to the neck muscles over time.

52: A: Physiology is the study of how the structure and systems of the body work together. Choice *B* refers to the definition of anatomy. Choices *C* and *D* are examples of physiology, but are not the definition of the term.

53. C: Systole, also referred to as systolic pressure, is correct because it is the required force to pump blood out of the heart. Choice *A*, blood pressure, is incorrect because that refers to the overall pressure of blood against the walls of blood vessels. Choice *B*, atherosclerosis, is incorrect because that is a medical condition where plaque builds up within the walls of an artery. Choice *D*, hypertension, is incorrect because it is a medical condition in which a person has abnormally high blood pressure.

54. C: Eversion is the correct answer because that refers to when the sole is rotated away from the midline of the body. Choice *A*, inversion, is incorrect because that is when the sole of the foot is moved toward the midline of the body. Choice *B*, pronation, is incorrect because it is an inward-rolling motion used to describe the movement of the arms, hands, and feet. Choice *D*, supination, is incorrect because it is an outward-rotating movement of the arms, hands, or feet.

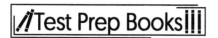
55. A: A dowager's hump often results from a forward head posture, often seen in people who spend a lot of time bent over a computer or working at office/desk jobs. Choice *B* is incorrect and does not refer to a dowager's hump. Choice *C* is a treatment for kyphosis, which causes a dowager's hump. Choice *D* refers to an anterior tilt in the pelvis.

56. B: An injury to the foot, knee, ankle, or pelvis can cause the client to favor the injured side and lean more heavily to the other side, causing an antalgic gait. An ataxic gait, Choice *A*, results from neurological problems. Choice *C*, an arthrogenic gait, is usually caused by osteoarthritis or rheumatoid arthritis, and a lurching gait, Choice *D*, is caused by weakness in the glutes.

57. A: Massage therapists should avoid wearing nail polish because it can harbor bacteria, which can give the client an infection. Whether or not nail polish is unattractive or unprofessional, Choices *B* and *C*, is a matter of personal opinion, and while it is not against any particular code of conduct, as in Choice *D*, it could potentially be against office or practice policies.

58. A: Sexual misconduct, including making unwanted sexual advances, is inappropriate and intolerable in a professional relationship. If a therapist makes sexual advances toward a client, the therapist should be dismissed from the practice immediately. Choice *B* is incorrect, as the situation is not the client's fault in any way. While some version of Choices *C* and *D* may be appropriate, those options should be up to the client after the therapist has been removed from the practice.

59. A: Multiple sclerosis is a condition where the myelin sheaths of the central nervous system neurons are destroyed. Choice *B*, Parkinson's disease, is incorrect because Parkinson's is a brain disorder that results in uncontrollable movement. Choice *C*, dementia, is incorrect because that is a general term for an impaired ability to think and remember. Choice *D*, Alzheimer's disease, is incorrect because it is a specific disease characterized by the destruction of brain cell connections, which results in memory impairment.

60. C: Trendelenburg's sign refers to when the hip on the affected side drops down during the stance phase of the gait. This gait is known as Trendelenburg gait. Choices *A* and *B* are made-up answers that are incorrect and do not refer to Trendelenburg's gait or sign, while Choice *D* is the opposite of the correct answer.

61. B: SOAP stands for subjective observations, objective observations, assessment, and plan. Choices *A*, *C*, and *D* are made-up answers.

62. D: Serotonin increases feelings of happiness and well-being. Choice *A*, oxytocin, is the "love hormone," which helps people create bonds with each other. Dopamine, Choice *B*, is responsible for pleasure and motivation, and Choice *C*, cortisol, is a hormone that can cause muscle tightness and tension.

63. A: Transference is when a client develops feelings for the therapist outside of a professional relationship. Massage therapy can be a very intimate process, both physically and emotionally, which can lead vulnerable clients to develop feelings for their therapist that are not based on the therapist-client relationship. Choice *B* is the opposite of transference and is called countertransference. Choices *C* and *D* are made-up answers.

64. C: Tetanus is the correct answer because it is a disease caused by the bacteria Clostridium tetani. The bacteria produce a toxin that results in muscle contractions, and the condition is characterized by

162

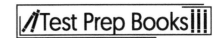

lockjaw, which is when the muscles of the neck and jaw lock up. Choice *A*, malaria, is incorrect because that is a parasitic infection that attacks red blood cells. Choice *B*, psoriasis, is incorrect because psoriasis is a skin disease that causes itchy rashes all over the skin. Choice *D*, tuberculosis, is incorrect because that is a bacterial disease that primarily affects the lungs.

65. D: Short, tight hip adductors often result in a scissors gait, which is commonly seen in cerebral palsy patients. Osteoarthritis, Choice *A*, typically causes an arthrogenic gait, while Parkinson's, Choice *C*, is typically characterized by short, shuffling steps. Choice *B*, diabetes, does not usually affect a client's gait.

66. C: Craniosacral therapy works with the flow of cerebrospinal fluid to provide health benefits to the client. While most types of massage can assist with the flow of blood and oxygen to the body and can affect the energy of the client both physically and emotionally, Choices *A*, *B*, and *D* are incorrect because they are not specifically the focus of craniosacral therapy.

67. A: A plumb line is a weighted length of string or wire suspended from the ceiling. It is used to make a visual assessment of a client's posture. Choices *B*, *C*, and *D* are made-up answers.

68. C: Estrogen levels are elevated during pregnancy and high levels of estrogen are known to increase the risk of forming blood clots. Choice *A*, luteinizing hormone, is incorrect because that is produced at lower rates during pregnancy. Choice *B*, aldosterone, is incorrect because aldosterone regulates salt and water levels in the kidneys and is not related to an increased risk of blood clots. Choice *D*, follicle stimulating hormone, is incorrect because its levels are considerably lower in pregnant females than non-pregnant females.

69. D: Wall angels are an exercise involving standing with the back and arms against the wall and bringing the elbows in towards the sides without lifting them off of the wall. Wall angels are used to bring relief to the pectoral muscles and rhomboids. Choices *A* and *B* are made-up, incorrect answers that do not refer to any exercises. Choice *C* refers to a stretch for the erector spinae in which the client lays on the floor with the buttocks against the wall and the leg stretched up the wall to create a 90-degree angle.

70. C: The parasympathetic nervous system controls the rest and digest functions and is part of the autonomic nervous system (ANS). Choice *B*, the fight-or-flight response, is controlled by the other branch of the ANS, the sympathetic nervous system. Choice *A* refers to bodily functions controlled by the brain, while Choice *D*, emotional responses, are controlled by the brain as well as chemicals such as hormones.

71. A: Acupuncture is a form of Eastern medicine that involves the use of needles placed at certain points in the body to help alleviate pain. Choice *B*, reflexology, involves massaging specific areas of the feet in order to soothe and treat other areas of the body. Cryotherapy, Choice *C*, is a branch of hydrotherapy that uses cold temperatures for treatment. Choice *D*, cupping, uses cups placed on the skin to create suction that can break up fascial adhesions.

72. C: SOAP refers to subjective, objective, assessment, and plan notes that a therapist makes about a client. SOAP notes can be particularly helpful for returning clients as a record of their ongoing treatment. Choices *A*, *B*, and *D* are made-up answers and are therefore incorrect.

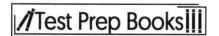

73. A: Massage therapists are obligated under HIPAA laws if they transmit medical information to third parties, making them a covered entity. Choices *B, C,* and *D* are incorrect; however, properly protecting a client's privacy should still be of the utmost importance.

74. D: Shiatsu massage involves the idea of controlling the body's energy flow along specific energy pathways. Swedish massage, Choice *A*, uses pressure and flowing movements to relax the body. Choice *B*, reflexology, works with pressure points in the feet to affect the rest of the body, and Choice *C*, Thai yoga massage, works the body through the use of passive stretching and compression.

75. B: Being late for an appointment and not making up the time is a service complaint. The therapist could lose their job if they do not provide clients with the amount of time for which they are scheduled. Choice *A* is an ethics violation. The therapist is not providing the standard nor quality of care to which they committed when they became licensed. Choice *C* is another ethics violation, which could result in the therapist losing their license to practice. Choice *D* is a frivolous complaint. Something caused the therapist to need to reschedule the appointment, which can be inconvenient, but the therapist made appropriate recompense by not only giving the client several days' notice of the cancellation but also by providing a discount for the rescheduled appointment.

76. C: Circumduction is a combination of several muscle movements that create a circular or cone-like movement. The shoulder and hip are both capable of circumduction. Choice *A*, rotation, is incorrect because it is when a limb moves about its long axis. Choice *B*, retraction, is incorrect because it is the movement of a body part in the posterior direction being drawn backwards. Choice *D*, protraction, is incorrect because it is the movement of a body part in the anterior position being drawn forward.

77. D: "It becomes less pliable" is the correct answer because with aging, the level of collagen in the body drops, making connective tissue become brittle and less pliable. Choice *A*, "it becomes discolored," is incorrect because the level of collagen decreasing does not affect the color of connective tissue. Choice *B*, "it is infected easily by pathogens," is incorrect because only a compromised immune system will make someone more susceptible to infection, and connective tissue is not a part of the immune system. Choice *C*, "it renews itself," is incorrect because eventually, with aging, connective tissue stops repairing itself.

78. D: Typically, only the client, the therapists, and the client's medical providers are authorized to view the client's medical records. The client can sometimes give other people, such as their spouse, immediate family, or a legal guardian, access to their records, as in Choices *A, B,* and *C*, but this is uncommon.

79. A: A client's diet is not a consideration in massage therapy. Choices *B, C,* and *D* are all part of the session. General and postural visual assessments and palpation assessments are done to determine the client's needs, while clinical reasoning is used to rule out contraindications, establish treatment goals, and evaluate the client's response to past treatments.

80. A: Mitochondria is an organelle within cells that oxidizes the end product of glycolysis, pyruvate, to produce the energy molecule ATP. Choice *B*, sarcomere, is incorrect because it is a structure that striated muscle is made out of. Sarcomeres consume chemical energy and do not produce it. Choice *C*, cytoplasm, is incorrect because it is the gelatinous liquid within cells where glycolysis occurs. Choice *D*, myocytes, is incorrect because they are muscle cells. Myocytes do contain a large quantity of mitochondria to produce the chemical energy needed to function.

81. B: Femoral nerve is the correct answer because it is superficial in the region of the inguinal triangle, a region of the groin near where the upper part of the leg meets the pubic area. This makes the inguinal triangle an endangerment site. Choice *A*, pelvic bone, is incorrect because it is deep within the area of the inguinal triangle and not a sensitive or easily damaged structure. Choice *C*, aortic arch, is incorrect because it resides within the chest cavity. Choice *D*, hippocampus, is incorrect because it is a structure of the limbic system in the brain.

82. B: It is important that the client feel comfortable during the intake process so they can disclose their medical problems or concerns as well as ask questions and discuss issues that may be of a sensitive nature. While the therapist may need to explain the services offered by the practice, Choice *A*, this is not part of the intake process. Similarly, it is not important that the client understand the laws and regulations of massage therapy, Choice *C*. Finally, the therapist is not a salesperson and should not be selling to the client, Choice *D*, during intake.

83. D: In addition to client privacy, HIPAA, the Health Insurance Portability and Accountability Act, also regulates record-keeping procedures and requirements. Practices may have their own rules regarding Choices *A*, *B*, and *C*, but those are not governed by HIPAA.

84. C: The circulatory system transports oxygenated erythrocytes (red blood cells) and other nutrients to cells to nourish them, so Choice *C* is correct. Choice *A*, respiratory system, is incorrect because this system is responsible for exchanging gases between the body and environment through breathing. Choice *B*, lymphatic system, is incorrect because the lymphatic system maintains body fluid levels and aids the immune system. Choice *D*, integumentary system, is incorrect because that is composed of the skin and its appendages and acts as a physical barrier protecting the inside of the body.

85. A: The stance phase is when the foot is making contact with the ground, and the swing phase is when the foot and leg are in the air. Choice *B* has the correct terms reversed, and Choices *C* and *D* are not the correct terms for the phases of the gait.

86. B: A therapist who works on a friend, relative, or business associate is involved in a dual relationship. While not a violation of ethics guidelines, Choice *A*, dual relationships can cause problems for both parties and are generally not advised. Transference and countertransference, Choices *C* and *D*, refer to personal feelings that develop after a therapist and client begin a massage therapy relationship.

87. D: The primary goal of oncology massage is to help the client relax and relieve the stress and anxiety of their cancer medications and treatments. Choice *A* refers to one of the key benefits of prenatal/pregnancy massage. Choice *B* refers to reflexology, and Choice *C* refers to Thai yoga massage.

88. C: The sciatic nerve runs from the lower back through the back of the thigh and down the lateral shins. Choice *A*, the femoral nerve, is the main nerve that runs through the tissue of the thigh and leg. The lateral plantar nerve, Choice *B*, is part of the toes. Choice *D*, the peroneal nerve, is the lower part of the sciatic nerve.

89. B: The relaxation phase occurs when calcium ions, ATP, ADP, or ATPase are unavailable for use. This phase can also be triggered when acetylcholine is released by a motor neuron. Choice *A*, latent period, is incorrect because it happens when calcium ions are released from the sarcoplasmic reticulum from an action potential being propagated along the sarcolemma. Choice *C*, excitation-contraction coupling phase, is incorrect because it refers to the overall process of electrical signals that initiates the release of calcium ions. Choice *D*, ATP hydrolysis phase, is incorrect because ATP hydrolysis is the process of ATP

165

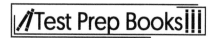
being used, changing it into ADP and a phosphate. This occurs just before actin is pulled for the muscle movement.

90. D: Acromial is the term related to the area of the body, at the shoulder, where the acromion bone is located. The acromion is the bony process of the scapula at the shoulder. Choice *A*, axillary, is incorrect because that refers to the side region of the body, including the armpit. Choice *B*, brachial, is incorrect because that refers to the region of the upper arm where the brachial artery and brachial plexus are located. Choice *C*, carpal, is incorrect because it is the region of the wrist where the carpal bones reside.

91. B: If the client is unable to clearly express an issue during a session, the therapist can help by asking relevant questions, such as "Does this hurt?" or "Is this the worst spot?" The therapist should never work a general area or try to guess where to focus the therapy, as in Choice *A*. In addition, the therapist should have already read over the client's records prior to the session, Choice *C*, and while asking another therapist for their professional opinion can be helpful, Choice *D*, it should not be done in the presence of the client.

92: C: Deep tissue massage has a number of contraindications, including Choices *A*, *B*, and *D*, so those choices are incorrect. While there are specific massage techniques for prenatal clients, pregnancy is not a specific contraindication of deep tissue massage.

93. A: Proprioception refers to the body's sense of limb position and orientation in space. Choices *B*, *C*, and *D* refer to the spinal nerves, the meninges, and the action potentials, respectively.

94. C: E-stim involves the application of a gentle electric current that stimulates specific muscles after an injury. Choice *A* refers to Esalen. Choice *B* refers to hot stone massage, and Choice *D* refers to hydrotherapy.

95. C: The CDC has established a set of standard precautions used to help limit the spread of infection. These include frequent hand-washing and changing sheets and towels between clients. Choices *A*, *B*, and *D* are made-up answers.

96. C: While the therapist should be aware of any medical conditions that affect the massage therapy, the therapist is not responsible for diagnosis. If the therapist suspects a possible medical issue, they should notify the client and suggest the client see an appropriate doctor. Choices *A*, *B*, and *D* are all part of the therapeutic relationship between therapist and client.

97. A: Varicose veins are considered a local contraindication, which is a condition in which a therapist is able to massage as long as they avoid an affected area. Choice *B*, neuritis, is incorrect because it is a total contraindication, meaning that massage should not be done due to the condition. Choice *C*, diabetes, is incorrect because it is a medical contraindication, which means that massage should only be done if a physician has approved of it beforehand. Choice *D*, cancer, is incorrect because it is also a condition that is a medical contraindication.

98. D: Soft lighting and relaxing music promote relaxation during a massage session. A massage therapy practice should always be clean and neat, Choice *A*, and a well-appointed office can promote professionalism, Choice *C*, but these are not relevant to the idea of stress reduction. While Choice *B* can be fun for employees, it would not create an environment that promotes relaxation for the client.

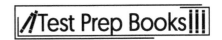

99. A: Kidney is the correct answer because it is not a portion of the alimentary canal, but an organ that filters blood and creates urine. The alimentary canal is the passageway for food through the body, starting at the mouth and ending with the anus. Choice *B*, mouth, is incorrect because that is the first portion of the alimentary canal. Choice *C*, rectum, is incorrect because that is the last portion of the alimentary canal before the anus. Choice *D*, pharynx, is incorrect because it is the second section of the alimentary canal after the mouth.

100. A: Gas exchange is the correct answer because the alveoli are sacs that fill with air inside the lungs, and their purpose is to add oxygen to blood and remove carbon dioxide from it. Choice *B*, blood filtration, is incorrect because waste in blood is filtered out by nephrons within the kidneys. Choice *C*, fluid transport, is incorrect because fluid transport is carried out by tube-like vessels, such as blood and lymphatic vessels. Choice *D*, antibody production, is incorrect because antibodies are produced by specialized white blood cells known as B lymphocytes.

Practice Test #3

1. Functional medicine is a Western style of medicine that focuses on the patient's:
    a. Spine and posture
    b. Ability to manage daily activities
    c. Range of motion
    d. Diet

2. Which of the following conditions requires a physician's approval before a massage can take place?
    a. Osteoporosis
    b. Sunburn
    c. Cuts
    d. Fever

3. Which forearm bone remains stationary when the wrist rotates?
    a. Radius
    b. Tibia
    c. Humerus
    d. Ulna

4. Which of the following are some contraindications of shiatsu massage?
    a. Preeclampsia, severe high blood pressure
    b. Bruises, recent surgery, tumors, inflamed skin
    c. Sunburn, varicose veins, warts, open wounds
    d. Contagious skin conditions, viruses

5. What might be used to assess a client's posture and gait?
    a. Visual observation of the client entering and leaving the office
    b. Having the client stand with feet together and bend over at the waist
    c. Measuring the length of the legs
    d. Anatomic landmarks such as the ears, clavicles, and pelvis

6. Which of the following is NOT a fungal infection?
    a. Pediculosis
    b. Ringworm
    c. Athlete's foot
    d. Candidiasis

7. Where would one find the lungs?
    a. Pleural cavity
    b. Pericardial cavity
    c. Pelvic cavity
    d. Abdominal cavity

8. The scapula is moved in a downward direction. What is this movement known as?
   a. Depression
   b. Adduction
   c. Elevation
   d. Abduction

9. What causes the erector spinae muscles to become hypertonic with regards to posture?
   a. Repetitive side-to-side movements
   b. Posterior head posture
   c. Forward head posture
   d. Hunched shoulders

10. How does trigger point therapy help to treat old injuries?
   a. It triggers the release of dopamine, which causes the brain to translate pain at the injury site into feelings of pleasure.
   b. Putting pressure on certain points in the feet helps to stimulate balance and healing in other areas of the body.
   c. The therapist uses finger pressure to combine pressure and stretching to stimulate the flow of energy in the body.
   d. It triggers nociceptors at the site of the injury, causing the brain to respond and increase blood flow to the area.

11. What structure is NOT involved in a reflex arc?
   a. Brainstem
   b. Spinal cord
   c. Receptor
   d. Motor neuron

12. What are the three phases of the therapist-client relationship?
   a. Pre-service, service, post-service
   b. Intake, treatment, close-out
   c. Pre-service, treatment, close-out
   d. Intake, service, post-service

13. What does inflammation of the iliotibial tract cause?
   a. Neck pain
   b. Abdominal pain
   c. Shoulder pain
   d. Knee pain

14. Which movement makes the angle between the sole of the foot and the back of the leg larger?
   a. Dorsiflexion
   b. Plantar flexion
   c. Pronation
   d. Adduction

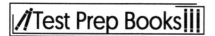

15. When a disease has no known cause, what terms is used?
    a. Congenital
    b. Epidemic
    c. Degenerative
    d. Idiopathic

16. What does a HIPAA release form indicate?
    a. Who can perform medical services on behalf of the patient
    b. Who can receive medical information about the patient
    c. Who can provide insurance coverage for the patient
    d. Who can discuss care options with the patient

17. Which type of muscle use results in a dynamic movement done at a constant velocity?
    a. Isokinetic muscle action
    b. Isometric contraction
    c. Resisted extension
    d. Concentric contraction

18. Where does the iliocostalis thoracis insert?
    a. Axis
    b. Occipital bone
    c. Upper six ribs
    d. Lower six ribs

19. Which of the following is responsible for the body's fight-or-flight response?
    a. Sympathetic nervous system
    b. Parasympathetic nervous system
    c. Autonomic nervous system
    d. Peripheral nervous system

20. Massage can increase the flow of fluids throughout the body and can be particularly helpful to the circulatory system. However, this can be dangerous for clients with which medical condition?
    a. Hypertension
    b. Diabetes
    c. Cancer
    d. New injury

21. How much time should a massage therapist allow between sessions in order to rest and prepare for the next client?
    a. Forty-five minutes
    b. Five minutes
    c. Thirty minutes
    d. Fifteen minutes

22. What does AMTA stand for?
    a. Association of Massage Therapists and Affiliates
    b. American Massage Therapists and Affiliates
    c. American Massage Therapy Association
    d. Affiliation of Massage Therapy Associates

23. What are ethics?
    a. A set of rules governing appropriate behavior
    b. Legal requirements for working in the massage therapy industry
    c. Guidelines specifying appropriate massage therapy techniques
    d. Rules for acceptable business administration practices

24. A person was in a car accident with a rapid acceleration then deceleration of the cervical vertebrae, resulting in neck pain, shoulder pain, and dizziness. What is the correct term for this injury?
    a. Neck sprain
    b. Herniated disk
    c. Whiplash
    d. Kyphosis

25. A person has an allergic reaction that results in localized swelling that is not systemically spreading. What is this known as?
    a. Atherosclerosis
    b. Angioedema
    c. Tuberculosis
    d. Psoriasis

26. What nerve is a distal branch off of the sciatic nerve?
    a. Digital nerve
    b. Supraclavicular nerve
    c. Radial nerve
    d. Tibial nerve

27. A person has a rip in their abdominal wall, resulting in a portion of their intestines pushing through and forming a bulge near the pubic area. What condition do they have?
    a. Abdominal aortic aneurysm
    b. Inguinal hernia
    c. Intraperitoneal hemorrhage
    d. Peritonitis

28. Which of the following is NOT a benefit of massage therapy for elderly clients?
    a. A chance to reconnect with their bodies
    b. Relief of aches and pains
    c. Stimulation of positive feelings from physical touch
    d. Relief from the discomfort of muscle growth and weight loss or gain

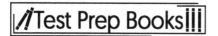

29. The phrase "out-of-pocket maximum" refers to
    a. The maximum amount that an insurance company will pay on behalf of a client
    b. The maximum a massage therapist can charge a client for a session
    c. The maximum number of massage therapy sessions a client can receive in a given year
    d. The maximum amount of money a patient will have to pay in a given year

30. What does NCBTMB stand for?
    a. National Certification Board for Therapy, Massage, and Bodywork
    b. National Classification Board for Therapeutic Massage and Bodywork
    c. National Certification Board for Therapeutic Massage and Bodywork
    d. National Certification Body for Therapy, Massage, and Bodywork

31. A high-pressured massage over a vascular structure can cause plaque to break loose and lodge in one location, almost entirely blocking a bloodstream. This is known as what?
    a. Thrombus
    b. Embolism
    c. Stroke
    d. Arrhythmia

32. A person has painful ureter contractions caused by crystals. What is this condition known as?
    a. Urinary tract infection
    b. Diabetes
    c. Renal colic
    d. Kidney disease

33. Which plane divides the body into anterior and posterior?
    a. The transverse plane
    b. The sagittal plane
    c. The coronal plane
    d. The mid-sagittal plane

34. Which classification of joint is the pubic symphysis?
    a. Cartilaginous joint
    b. Fibrous joint
    c. Synovial joint
    d. Plane joint

35. What is isometric contraction?
    a. Muscle contraction via manual manipulation
    b. Muscle contraction involving passive resistance
    c. Muscle contraction via autonomous manipulation
    d. Muscle contraction involving active resistance

36. A complex chemical is built up from simpler molecules. What is this process known as?
    a. Metabolism
    b. Catabolism
    c. Differentiation
    d. Anabolism

172

37. A massage therapist provides therapy services to their spouse. This is what type of violation?
    a. A dual relationship violation
    b. A transference violation
    c. A HIPAA violation
    d. This is not a violation.

38. What is the difference between acute pain and chronic pain?
    a. Acute pain is sharp and stabbing, while chronic pain is dull and throbbing.
    b. Acute pain is dull and throbbing, while chronic pain is sharp and stabbing.
    c. Chronic pain comes on quickly, while acute pain is long-lasting.
    d. Acute pain comes on quickly, while chronic pain is long-lasting.

39. A massage therapist does three massages at a billing rate of $100 per massage. The therapist is paid 50% of the revenue, or $150 for the work. What type of payment is the therapist likely receiving?
    a. Commission
    b. Salary
    c. Independent contractor income
    d. W2 income

40. What does the peripheral/central/peripheral massage protocol involve?
    a. Working the limbs from the heart outward
    b. Working the entire torso or large muscle area before focusing on the specific target area
    c. Working through massage on the entire body before focusing on specific areas
    d. Working with light pressure before moving on to deep-tissue work

41. The connection between a patients' calf muscle and heel bone was severed. Which type of structure was damaged?
    a. Ligament
    b. Bone
    c. Muscle
    d. Tendon

42. Which of the following is NOT one of the roles of the state licensing boards?
    a. Making legislative changes
    b. Creating and enforcing disciplinary policies
    c. Updating rules and regulations for the field
    d. Providing salary and insurance information

43. What are finger cots?
    a. Medical devices that provide support to strengthen weakened fingers
    b. Fitted pressure gloves that reduce swelling in aching fingers
    c. Protective latex coverings for the fingertips rather than the whole hand
    d. Attachments to the massage table where a client can rest their hands

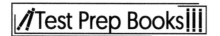

44. What does PRICE involve?
  a. Pressure, Rest, Ice, Compression, and Elevation
  b. Protection, Relaxation, Ice, Compression, and Elevation
  c. Protection, Rest, Ice, Compression, and Elevation
  d. Protection, Rest, Isolation, Compression, and Elevation

45. Where would one find the stratum lucidum?
  a. Brain
  b. Eyes
  c. Hands
  d. Hair

46. What do trigger points feel like upon palpation?
  a. Smooth and yielding
  b. Warm to the touch
  c. Pliable and easily maneuvered
  d. Textured, like pebbles beneath the surface of the skin

47. A person has a condition where their antibodies attack their own tissues. What is this condition known as?
  a. Lymphoma
  b. Human immunodeficiency virus
  c. Encephalitis
  d. Lupus

48. Manual therapy is often measured and billed in what increments?
  a. Ten to fifteen minutes
  b. Five minutes
  c. Twenty to thirty minutes
  d. Forty-five minutes

49. Swollen glands are a contraindication for massage and are likely due to which issue?
  a. Compromised immune system
  b. Infection
  c. Muscle sprain
  d. Nerve damage

50. What should be used at the beginning of every massage?
  a. Stretching
  b. Stillness
  c. Warming up
  d. Cooling down

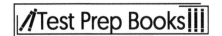

51. What course of action should be taken if a client makes an unwanted sexual advance towards the therapist?
    a. The relationship should be terminated and the client should be removed from the practice.
    b. The therapist should be dismissed from the practice for not keeping the client in line in a professional way.
    c. The client should be assigned to another therapist.
    d. The manager should take over the client's care.

52. Which muscles are primarily responsible for extending the leg?
    a. Quadriceps femoris
    b. Gastrocnemius
    c. Soleus
    d. Tibialis anterior

53. A style of medicine that focuses on the client's entire self rather than only on a specific area is called
    a. Holistic medicine
    b. Eastern medicine
    c. Hydrotherapy
    d. Physical therapy

54. What information should be included under the subjective section of the SOAP notes?
    a. Client complaints, such as pain, headaches, or insomnia
    b. Tests and assessment of the client's posture, gait, and motion
    c. The procedures and techniques performed
    d. Strategies for continued care, such as stretches or self-care exercises

55. Which structure blocks the airway when one swallows?
    a. Larynx
    b. Epiglottis
    c. Cricoid cartilage
    d. Laryngeal prominence

56. Extrapyramidal symptoms can occur as a result of what?
    a. Developing dementia
    b. Kidney failure
    c. Taking antipsychotic drugs
    d. Strenuous muscle use

57. What is NOT a benefit of communication at the end of a client's session?
    a. The therapist can answer any questions the client has about their treatment.
    b. The therapist can suggest how the client can maintain or extend the benefits of the massage.
    c. The therapist can provide recommendations for stretches, other services, or referrals the client may need.
    d. The therapist and client can engage in personal conversation to deepen their relationship.

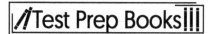

58. When moving the ankle, which muscle is a synergist to the soleus?
    a. Pronator teres
    b. Flexor carpi radialis
    c. Sternocleidomastoid
    d. Gastrocnemius

59. An anthrogenic gait is often caused by:
    a. A weak or misfiring gluteus medius muscle
    b. Osteoarthritis or rheumatoid arthritis in the hip, knee, or ankle joints
    c. An injury to the foot, ankle, knee, or pelvis
    d. Neurological problems, such as a lack of balance or muscle coordination

60. Why is hydration especially important for athletes?
    a. It helps normalize blood pressure.
    b. It helps prevent cramping and muscle spasms.
    c. It helps flush bacteria from the body.
    d. It helps regulate body temperature.

61. Which term describes a region of the body where veins, arteries, and nerves lie close to the surface of the body?
    a. Areas of edema
    b. Local contraindication
    c. Endangerment site
    d. Trauma site

62. A technique used to elongate joints or lengthen the torso or a limb is called:
    a. Stretching
    b. Trigger point therapy
    c. Traction
    d. Joint mobilization

63. Which massage technique incorporates a series of assisted yoga positions?
    a. Swedish massage
    b. Sports massage
    c. Thai massage
    d. Prenatal massage

64. Pitted edema can indicate what serious condition(s)?
    a. Cardiovascular or kidney dysfunction
    b. Contusions and hematomas
    c. Varicose veins
    d. Embolism

65. What does the acronym ROM stand for?
    a. Range of movement
    b. Rotation of movement
    c. Range of motion
    d. Rotation of motion

66. Which term best describes muscle spindles?
    a. Tropomyosin
    b. Proprioceptors
    c. Sarcoplasm
    d. Myocytes

67. Which foramen is located in the pelvis?
    a. Ethmoid
    b. Lacerum
    c. Obturator
    d. Intervertebral

68. What is a dual relationship?
    a. When the therapist also acts as a counselor to a client
    b. When the therapist has a personal relationship with a client
    c. When the therapist is also the manager of the practice
    d. When the therapist has a second job outside of massage therapy

69. What is palpation?
    a. The use of touch to identify a specific muscle or anatomical structure
    b. The use of a kneading technique to perform deep tissue massage
    c. The use of a gliding stroke with constant pressure during treatment
    d. A percussive technique using quick, well-aimed strokes

70. The health history form includes all of the following information EXCEPT:
    a. Therapist preference
    b. Types of services
    c. Medical history and health conditions
    d. Preferred techniques or modalities

71. Which medical issue is due to a bacterial infection?
    a. Herpes
    b. Shingles
    c. Plantar warts
    d. Boils

72. What should a therapist do if they have a contradicting or alternate opinion on a doctor's determination for a client's prescribed treatment plan?
    a. Tell the client that their doctor may not be very good and suggest getting a second opinion.
    b. Explain the benefits of the therapist's approach and suggest further research for the client.
    c. Tell the client anecdotes that the therapist has heard about the doctor and suggest that they should find a new doctor for treatment.
    d. Explain that the doctor's treatment plan is incorrect and detail better treatment options for the client.

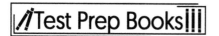
73. Which of the following is NOT an example of homeostatic regulation?
    a. Parathyroid releasing hormones when calcium levels are too low
    b. Shivering in cold weather
    c. Hair regrowing after being pulled out
    d. Sweat glands producing sweat when exposed to heat

74. Which body system involves the pituitary gland?
    a. Circulatory
    b. Nervous
    c. Endocrine
    d. Integumentary

75. The muscle energy technique (MET) is a form of stretching tailored to which particular group of clients?
    a. Athletes
    b. Pregnant women
    c. Elderly clients
    d. Oncology patients

76. What is the main principle and physical benefit of massage therapy?
    a. Reducing tension throughout the body
    b. Increasing muscle flexibility
    c. Increasing circulation
    d. Reducing the client's stress levels

77. Which is NOT a consideration in proper body mechanics for a massage therapist?
    a. Proper posture
    b. Correct table height
    c. Taking short breaks to rest the hands and arms
    d. Correct hand and arm techniques

78. What pertinent information is NOT required for oncology massage?
    a. The client's dietary restrictions
    b. The client's type of cancer
    c. Details about the client's blood work
    d. The status of the client's lymph nodes

79. What is lordosis?
    a. An anterior tilt in the client's pelvis
    b. A stoop or hump-like posture
    c. A severe curvature of the spine
    d. An exercise involving contracting the glutes while in a knees-bent, supine posture

178

80. What is craniosacral therapy?
    a. The study of how the structures and systems of the body work together
    b. The use of gliding strokes to apply constant pressure to the scalp and neck during therapy
    c. A ten- to twenty-minute massage that works the upper posterior body, neck, and arms
    d. A form of bodywork that uses touch to manipulate the synarthrodial joints according to the subtle rhythms of living tissue

81. A massage therapist stops a therapy session to take a personal phone call. This is an example of a(n)
    a. Ethics violation
    b. Service violation
    c. Provider-patient confidentiality
    d. HIPAA violation

82. Which hormone is referred to as the "love hormone"?
    a. Serotonin
    b. Dopamine
    c. Oxytocin
    d. Cortisol

83. When in the anatomical position, which statement is true?
    a. The palms are facing backwards.
    b. The body is lying down with the face up.
    c. Feet are flat and directed to the sides.
    d. The thumb is on the lateral side of the hand.

84. Drop foot is often an indication of:
    a. Cerebrovascular incident (such as a stroke)
    b. Neurological and/or muscular issues
    c. Long periods of immobilization
    d. Short, tight hip adductors

85. Why is it unacceptable to send SOAP notes in the body of an email sent to another therapist?
    a. HIPAA regulations prohibit sharing client information with other therapists.
    b. Client privacy is not protected when sending information in the body of an email.
    c. The client must personally share their medical records.
    d. SOAP notes do not provide enough information for another therapist to understand the client's medical needs.

86. Adjustment involves the release of gas that builds up in the joints due to injury, poor posture, or daily wear and tear. What type of practitioner typically provides adjustments for clients?
    a. An aromatherapist
    b. A chiropractor
    c. A reflexologist
    d. An esthetician

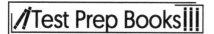

87. When in the sitting position, which structure supports the body?
    a. Deltoid tuberosity
    b. Greater trochanter
    c. Calcaneum
    d. Ischial tuberosity

88. What is a contraindication?
    a. A medication that the client takes that could affect the success of massage therapy
    b. A particular massage therapy that would be specifically helpful to a client
    c. A medical issue that precludes a client from receiving a service
    d. A medical condition for which massage therapy is specifically prescribed

89. Where is the anterior scalene muscle located?
    a. Abdomen
    b. Head
    c. Neck
    d. Back

90. What does the cross-fiber friction technique involve?
    a. Rubbing muscle fibers perpendicular to the grain
    b. Massaging muscle fibers along the grain
    c. Soft massage using the effleurage technique
    d. Kneading the muscle using the petrissage technique

91. What is the purpose of an insurance claim?
    a. It notifies the insurance company that a client has been injured.
    b. The therapist uses it to bill the client's insurance company for the services performed.
    c. It allows the insurance company to bill the service provider on behalf of the client.
    d. The client uses it to submit a HIPAA authorization to the insurance company.

92. Which is an example of countertransference?
    a. The therapist recommends that the client see a doctor to address a particular medical issue.
    b. The therapist determines that the client needs additional therapy sessions to fully address their massage needs.
    c. The therapist learns that the client has the same breed of dog and invites the client to bring their dog to a "play date" at the local dog park.
    d. The client becomes attracted to the therapist and asks the therapist out on a date.

93. Which type of massage stroke is a quick, percussive technique?
    a. Tapotement
    b. Effleurage
    c. Petrissage
    d. Touch

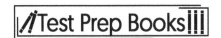

94. A massage therapist working in an office with a chiropractor and a physical therapist keeps their patient files in a large filing cabinet along the back wall of their office in the practice. Is this a HIPAA violation?
    a. Yes, because the filing cabinet containing patient records must be locked.
    b. Yes, because the filing cabinet must be located in a private, locked room.
    c. No, because massage therapists are not covered entities under HIPAA.
    d. No, because the records are stored away from other patients and medical professionals in the practice.

95. A person has a large amount of fluid building up in their interstitial tissue spaces. Which of the following is most likely the issue?
    a. Edema
    b. Allergies
    c. Lymphoma
    d. Cellulitis

96. Which of the following is NOT a benefit of specialization?
    a. Targeting a particular demographic to gain clients
    b. Honing specific skills in a particular style of therapy
    c. Building a private practice focused on a particular clientele
    d. Developing a broad range of knowledge in a variety of treatment options

97. What is the purpose of cold therapy in massage?
    a. Treats chronic issues
    b. Stimulates inflammation to relax locked muscles
    c. Controls initial pain and reduces swelling
    d. Increases blood flow, providing oxygen and nutrients to the area

98. What does the phrase "scope of practice" mean?
    a. What a professional is and is not allowed to do within a work setting
    b. What services and therapies are provided by the practice
    c. How many employees the practice can have
    d. The types of procedures a therapist is licensed to perform

99. What is a common cause of kyphosis?
    a. Hyperextending a joint during exercise
    b. Carrying a heavy baby during pregnancy
    c. Spending too much time bent over a computer or desk
    d. Repetitive movements from activities such as typing

100. What is the most superior region of the vertebral column?
    a. Cervical
    b. Sacral
    c. Lumbar
    d. Thoracic

Answer Explanations #3

1. D: Functional medicine focuses mainly on the patient's diet and is often used to treat gastrointestinal conditions like IBS and Crohn's disease. Choices *A, B*, and *C* are incorrect.

2. A: Osteoporosis is the correct answer because it results in bones becoming weak and brittle, and is an example of a medical contraindication. Therefore, it requires a physician's approval for massage to occur. Choices *B* and *C*, sunburn and cuts, are incorrect because they are local contraindications, meaning that massage can occur as long as the affected area is avoided. Choice *D*, fever, is incorrect because it is a total contraindication, meaning that massage should be completely avoided for clients with a fever.

3. D: Ulna is the correct answer because when the wrist rotates, the head of the radius pivots, while the ulna does not move. Choice *A*, radius, is incorrect because the radius is the forearm bone that rotates during wrist movements. Choice B, tibia, is incorrect because the tibia is located in the lower leg, not the forearm. Choice *C*, humerus, is incorrect because that is the bone of the upper arm.

4. B: Bruises, inflamed skin, tumors, and recent surgeries are some of the contraindications of shiatsu massage. Choice *A* lists contraindications of prenatal massage, and Choices *C* and *D* both refer to reflexology.

5. D: The therapist can use anatomic landmarks such as the ears, clavicles, hands, and pelvis to make a visual assessment of the client's posture and gait. While visual observations listed in Choice *A* might show obvious issues, such as a defined limp, an assessment should be conducted in a more controlled way. Choices *B* and *C* refer to specific tests to evaluate the possibility of scoliosis and are usually performed by a physician.

6. A: Pediculosis is the correct answer because it is a lice infestation, which is considered parasitic. Choice *B*, ringworm, is incorrect because ringworm is a skin infection caused by a fungus. Up to forty different types of fungi may cause a ringworm rash. Choice *C*, athlete's foot, is incorrect because that is a fungal skin infection that typically originates between toes and is due to the same type of fungi as ringworm. Choice *D*, candidiasis, is incorrect because that is a fungal infection of the skin or mucous membranes. Candidiasis is more commonly known as a yeast infection.

7. A: The pleural cavity is within the thoracic cavity, where the lungs are located. Choice *B*, pericardial cavity, is incorrect because that is a body cavity within the thoracic cavity that contains the heart. Choice *C*, pelvic cavity, is incorrect because that is the lowest ventral body cavity, located at the pelvis. Choice *D*, abdominal cavity, is incorrect because that is a lower ventral cavity, beneath the lungs, that contains the majority of the digestive tract, the liver, the kidney, and many other organs.

8. A: Depression is the correct answer because it describes the inferior movement of a body part. Choice *B*, adduction, is incorrect because it is the movement of a limb closer to the midline of the body. Choice *C*, elevation, is incorrect because it is an upward movement of a body part. Choice *D*, abduction, is incorrect because it is a movement of a limb away from the midline of the body.

9. C: Forward head posture causes the erector spinae muscles to become hypertonic due to the incorrect head position. Choices *A, B*, and *D* are made-up answers and therefore incorrect.

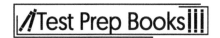

10. D: Trigger point therapy stimulates nociceptors at the injury site, which causes the brain to increase blood flow to that area. Choice *A* is incorrect, as dopamine is one of the pleasure hormones that does not come into play in trigger point therapy. Choice *B* refers to reflexology, and Choice *C* refers to shiatsu massage.

11. A: Brainstem is the correct answer because it is not involved in a reflex arc. A reflex arc speeds up reflex time by not involving the brain or brain stem. Choice *B*, spinal cord, is incorrect because in a reflex arc, information from sensory neurons is integrated in the interneurons of the spinal cord and then sent to motor neurons to respond to the stimulus. Choice *C*, receptor, is incorrect because receptors detect stimuli to initiate a reflex arc. Choice *D*, motor neuron, is incorrect because the motor neurons are the last portion of a reflex arc. They receive the information for the reflexive response to stimuli and then respond with an action.

12. D: The three phases of the therapist-client relationship are intake, service, and post-service. Choices *A*, *B*, and *C* are made-up answers.

13. D: The iliotibial tract runs along the lateral thigh from the iliac crest to the tibia. Inflammation of this tract can cause knee pain, particularly in runners and cyclists. Choices *A*, *B*, and *C* are incorrect.

14. A: Dorsiflexion is the movement of pointing the feet upward toward the shins, thus making the angle between the sole and the back of the leg greater. Choice *B*, plantar flexion, is incorrect because it is the opposite movement where the angle between the sole and the back of the leg becomes smaller. Choice *C*, pronation, is incorrect because that is an inward rotating motion. Choice *D*, adduction, is incorrect because that is a movement towards the body's midline, such as bringing the knees together.

15. D: Idiopathic refers to a disease with no known cause. Choice *A*, congenital, is incorrect because that refers to a condition that is present at birth. Choice *B*, epidemic, is incorrect because that is a widespread disease within a specific community. Choice *C*, degenerative, is incorrect because that refers to a progressive loss of function in organs as a result of a disease.

16. B: The HIPAA release form indicates who can receive medical information about the patient. Patients are often asked to sign a HIPAA release form when they visit doctor's offices and other medical providers. Choices *A*, *C*, and *D* are incorrect.

17. A: Isokinetic muscle actions are naturally occurring muscle contractions composed of movements at a constant velocity. Choice *B*, isometric contraction, is incorrect because that is when a muscle generates force while attempting to shorten. Choice *C*, resisted extension, is incorrect because that is a form of muscle movement with resistance against it. Therapists often use resisted muscle movements to detect or evaluate issues with muscle performance. Choice *D*, concentric contraction, is incorrect ecause concentric contraction is when a muscle's force is greater than a resistance applied.

18. C: The upper six ribs is the location where the iliocostalis thoracis muscle inserts. The iliocostalis thoracis originates from the lower six ribs. Choice *A*, axis, is incorrect because that is the insertion location for the spinalis cervicis muscle. Choice *B*, occipital bone, is incorrect because the occipital bone is the insertion location of the spinalis capitis muscle. Choice *D*, lower six ribs, is incorrect because that is where the iliocostalis lumborum inserts.

19. A: The sympathetic nervous system is responsible for the body's fight-or-flight response. The parasympathetic nervous system, Choice *B*, is responsible for rest-and-digest functions, and the

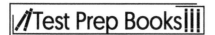

sympathetic and parasympathetic nervous systems together make up the autonomic nervous system, Choice *C*. Choice *D* refers to the nerves that are outside of the brain and spinal cord.

20. A: While increasing the body's circulation is beneficial for most clients, it can be dangerous for clients with hypertension. Some types of massage are contraindicated for diabetes, cancer, and fresh injuries as well, but Choices *B, C,* and *D* are incorrect here.

21. D: A fifteen-minute break between sessions allows the therapist to physically recover and reset the therapy room for the next client. While longer breaks, such as in Choices *A* and *C*, can be nice, too many long breaks can affect how many sessions a therapy can do and thus affect the therapist's earnings. Choice *B*, five minutes, is not enough time either to recover or to reset the room.

22. C: AMTA stands for the American Massage Therapy Association. Choices *A, B,* and *D* are all made-up names.

23. A: Ethics refer to the rules that govern appropriate behavior. They are not necessarily legal requirements, Choice *B*, though many ethics violations are also legal and/or licensing violations. Choice *C* is incorrect because, while ethics should be considered during a massage session, they do not dictate specific therapy techniques. Ethics should be considered in business administration practices, Choice *D*, but those practices are not the definition of ethics.

24. C: Whiplash is the correct answer because it is the result of the head moving suddenly backward and then forward. Choice *A*, neck sprain, is incorrect because that refers to when a muscle or ligament of the neck is stretched to a point where it is damaged. Choice *B*, herniated disk, is incorrect because that happens when a spinal disk bulges out of place, resulting in pain and limited motion. Choice *D*, kyphosis, is incorrect because that is an overly large curvature of the spine that is greater than fifty degrees.

24. B: Angioedema is swelling under skin that is the result of an allergic reaction. Choice *A*, atherosclerosis, is incorrect because that is an artery disease that causes plaque to build up within an artery and harden. Choice *C*, tuberculosis, is incorrect because tuberculosis is a bacterial respiratory disease caused by Mycobacterium tuberculosis. Choice *D*, psoriasis, is incorrect because that is a disease that causes itchy and scaly rashes on the skin.

26. D: Tibial nerve is the correct answer because the sciatic nerve extends from the hip down the leg towards the tibia. At the start of the tibia, the sciatic nerve branches into the tibial nerve and others. Choice *A*, digital nerve, is incorrect because the digital nerves are located in the fingers and branch from the median, ulnar, and radial nerves. Choice *B*, supraclavicular nerve, is incorrect because this nerve is located in the neck and branches from the third and fourth cervical nerves. Choice *C*, radial nerve, is incorrect because the radial nerve is located in the forearm and originates from a branch of the brachial plexus.

27. B: An inguinal hernia is a hole in the abdominal wall near the pubic area that results in a portion of the internal organs pushing through the hole. Choice *A*, abdominal aortic aneurysm, is incorrect because that is a weakening in the abdominal aorta that causes a bulge and has a high risk of rupturing. Choice *C*, intraperitoneal hemorrhage, is incorrect because that refers to internal bleeding within the peritoneal cavity in the abdomen. Choice *D*, peritonitis, is incorrect because peritonitis is an inflammation of the peritoneum in the abdomen.

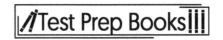

28. D: This choice refers to the benefits of massage for new mothers. Elderly clients can benefit from all of the positive aspects of massage mentioned in Choices *A, B,* and *C*.

29. D: The out-of-pocket maximum refers to the maximum amount of money a patient will be required to pay in a given year. Insurance policies often cover services at 100% once the patient's out-of-pocket maximum has been met. Choices *A, B,* and *C* are incorrect.

30. C: NCBTMB is the National Certification Board for Therapeutic Massage and Bodywork. Choices *A, B,* and *D* are made-up answers.

31. B: Embolism is the correct answer because it occurs when a blood clot breaks loose and lodges within a smaller vessel, largely restricting blood flow. Choice *A*, thrombus, is incorrect because that is the term for a blood clot that is lodged in place within a vascular vessel, impeding blood flow but not blocking it off. Choice *C*, stroke, is incorrect because that occurs when blood is blocked from going to the brain. Choice *D*, arrhythmia, is incorrect because arrhythmia is an irregular rhythm to a heartbeat.

32. C: Renal colic is the correct answer because that is what happens when a painful stone blocks a ureter. Choice *A*, urinary tract infection, is incorrect because that is an infection anywhere within the urinary system. Choice *B*, diabetes, is incorrect because diabetes is a disease that results in too much sugar in the blood. Choice *D*, kidney disease, is incorrect because that is a disease of the kidneys that leads to renal failure.

33. C: The coronal (or frontal) plane divides the body into anterior and posterior. The transverse plane, Choice *A*, divides the body into upper and lower halves, while the sagittal plane, Choice *B*, divides the body into right and left. Choice *D* is a made-up term, though the mid-sagittal line refers to the body's midline.

34. A: Cartilaginous joint is the correct answer because these joints are composed of two bones bound by cartilage and allow minimal movement. The pubic symphysis is a cartilaginous attachment of the left and right pelvic bones. Choice *B*, fibrous joint, is incorrect because these are joints connected by tough fibrous tissue that do not allow movement. The fibrous joints are found in the skull. Choice *C*, synovial joint, is incorrect because these are joints between two moving bones that are fluid-filled and contain articular cartilage. An example of a synovial joint is the elbow. Choice *D*, plane joint, is incorrect because a plane joint is a flat surface between bones that allow them to glide against each other. An example of a plane joint is a joint between the metacarpal bones.

35. B: Isometric contraction refers to muscle contraction involving passive resistance. Choice *D* substitutes "active" for "passive," making it incorrect. Choices *A* and *C* are incorrect and do not refer to isometric contraction.

36. D: Anabolism is the process of larger and more complex molecules forming from simpler components. Choice *A*, metabolism, is incorrect because metabolism is the entire sum of all anabolic and catabolic reactions within a body. Choice *B*, catabolism, is incorrect because that is the process of complex molecules breaking down into smaller molecules. Choice *C*, differentiation, is incorrect because that is the process of stem cells changing into cells with specialized functions.

37. D: A massage therapist can provide services to their spouse should they so choose, and it is not a violation of any laws or regulations. Having a dual relationship, Choice *A*, can sometimes be problematic, though it is not in direct violation of any legalities. Choice *B*, transference, refers to when a client

185

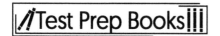
develops feelings for a therapist outside of the professional relationship, and Choice C refers to patient privacy laws and regulations.

38. D: Acute pain comes on quickly, often as a result of an injury or sudden stress on the body, such as from a fall or accident, or from sleeping in an uncomfortable position. Chronic pain is pain that lasts more than six weeks. Choices A and B refer to specific feelings of pain that are not directly related to the timeline of the pain. Choice C is incorrect, as the terms are reversed.

39. A: The therapist is likely being paid on commission, which is a percentage of the revenue for the services performed. Some employees are paid either a salary, Choice B, or an hourly rate, Choice D, both of which are reported on W2 forms. Independent contractors, Choice C, are paid their gross rate without the deduction of any taxes. An independent contractor can be paid on commission, but is not always paid this way.

40. B: The peripheral/central/peripheral protocol involves working with the torso or with the large muscles, massaging the entire area before narrowing the focus to the specific area of issue. Choice A refers to the proximal/distal/proximal technique, which is similar but involves the limbs. Choice C refers to the general/specific/general protocol, and Choice D refers to the superficial/deep/superficial protocol.

41. D: A tendon is a connective tissue that attaches muscle to bone. Choice A, ligament, is incorrect because a ligament attaches one bone to another bone to provide support and stability at joints. Choice B, bone, is incorrect because the purpose of bones is to give shape and provide structural support to the body, not to connect muscles to bones. Choice C, muscle, is incorrect because the only function of the muscles is to enable movement.

42. D: The state licensing boards make legislative changes, create and enforce disciplinary policies, and keep the rules and regulations for the field updated, making Choices A, B, and C incorrect. They do not provide salary or insurance information. Salary information can be found via sites such as Glassdoor, and insurance information can be found through organizations like the ABMP or AMTA.

43. C: Finger cots are protective latex coverings for the fingers. They cover only the fingers rather than the whole hand and can be a good alternative to gloves when protecting a cut or wound on the fingers. Choices A, B, and D are made-up answers.

44. C: PRICE is an acronym for Protection, Rest, Ice, Compression, and Elevation. Choices A, B, and D all include an incorrect word.

45. C: Hands is the correct answer because the stratum lucidum layer of the epidermis can be found in the skin of the palms, soles, and digits. The stratum lucidum is a thin translucent layer only found in thicker portions of the epidermis. Choice A, brain, is incorrect because it is composed of two major categories of tissue, grey matter and white matter, neither of which is an epidermis layer. Choice B, eyes, is incorrect because the eye is a complex organ made of many tissues, such as the sclera, cornea, and iris. They do not contain any epidermis layers. Choice D, hair, is incorrect because hair is composed of the protein actin and is not part of the epidermis.

46. D: Trigger points are described as feeling like pebbles beneath the skin. Choices A, B, and C all refer to healthy muscle tissue.

186

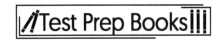

47. D: Lupus is a condition where antibodies attack a variety of their own body tissues. Choice *A*, lymphoma, is incorrect because lymphoma is a cancer of the lymph nodes. Choice *B*, human immunodeficiency virus, is incorrect because that is a virus that impairs the immune system. Choice *C*, encephalitis, is incorrect because that is inflammation of the brain.

48. A: Manual therapy is the term used to bill insurance for massage therapy work. It is usually measured in ten- to fifteen-minute increments. Choices *B, C,* and *D* are incorrect.

49. B: Infection is the correct answer because it can cause swollen glands and is often a contraindication for massage, as it can result in the spread of an infection. Choice *A*, compromised immune system, is incorrect because a compromised immune system may not result in swollen glands and is not a contraindication for massage. Choice *C*, muscle sprain, is incorrect because that occurs when a muscle is stretched too far. Choice *D*, nerve damage, is incorrect because it doesn't result in swollen glands, although it can cause lack of sensation.

50. B: Each massage session should begin with stillness, a few moments or quiet time of breathing deeply and relaxing before beginning the massage. Choice *A*, stretching, is involved in some types of massage, but not necessarily all of them. Choices *C* and *D* are more akin to working out than massage therapy.

51. A: If a client makes an unwanted sexual advance towards their therapist, the relationship should be terminated and the client should be removed from the practice. The client's behavior is not the fault of the therapist, so the therapist should not be punished as in Choice *B*. Should the client stay with either another therapist or the manager, that would make for a potentially uncomfortable environment, so Choices *C* and *D* are also incorrect.

52. A: Quadriceps femoris is the correct answer because the quadriceps femoris group is primarily responsible for a leg extension movement. Choice *B*, gastrocnemius, is incorrect because that is the primary calf muscle and is responsible for pulling the heel up and extending the foot downwards. Choice *C*, soleus, is incorrect because that is the other main calf muscle group that assists in plantarflexion. Choice *D*, tibialis anterior, is incorrect because that is a muscle in the shin of the leg that allows dorsiflexion of the foot.

53. A: Holistic medicine focuses on treating the client's whole self, as opposed to treating a particular illness, injury, or specific treatment area. While many types of holistic medicine, such as acupuncture, are Eastern in origin, as in Choice *B*, this isn't always the case. Choice *C*, hydrotherapy, refers to the use of temperature treatments, such as an ice pack or heating pad. Physical therapy, Choice *D*, refers to stretches and exercises that are prescribed to aid a client's healing.

54. A: The subjective section of the SOAP notes should include information about the client's concerns and priorities for the session, including any pain or issues the client is experiencing that need to be addressed. Choice *B* refers to the objective section of the notes, Choice *C* refers to the activity section, and Choice *D* refers to the plan section.

55. B: Epiglottis is the correct answer because it is a flap of cartilage at the back of the mouth that blocks the windpipe when one is swallowing. Choice *A*, larynx, is incorrect because the larynx is a muscular and cartilaginous organ beneath the epiglottis. Choice *C*, cricoid cartilage, is incorrect because that is the circular-shaped cartilage in the larynx that holds the airway open and attaches to the cricothyroid, lateral cricoarytenoid, and posterior cricoarytenoid muscles. Choice *D*, laryngeal prominence, is

187

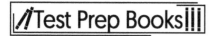
incorrect because that is a portion of the thyroid cartilage that covers the larynx. It protects the larynx and the vocal cords.

56. C: "Taking antipsychotic drugs" is the correct answer because extrapyramidal symptoms, such as tremors, stiff muscles, and involuntary movements, can be a side effect of antipsychotic drugs. Choice *A*, developing dementia, is incorrect because the results of dementia are forgetfulness, impaired thinking, and limited social skills. Choice *B*, kidney failure, is incorrect because there are many symptoms of kidney failure, such as fatigue, shortness of breath, fluid retention, and nausea. However, extrapyramidal symptoms are not a result of kidney failure. Choice *D*, strenuous exercise, is incorrect because that results in fatigue, shortness of breath, elevated heart rate, muscle soreness, and more.

57. D: The therapist should avoid personal conversation and relationships with a client, especially if the client's treatment is ongoing. Choices *A*, *B*, and *C* all represent benefits of communication with the client at the end of the client's session.

58. D: Gastrocnemius is the correct answer because, along with the soleus and plantaris, it is a calf muscle and plays a large role in foot and ankle movement. Choices *A* and *B*, pronator teres and flexor carpi radialis, are incorrect because they are muscles of the forearm that are responsible for wrist movements. Choice *C*, sternocleidomastoid, is incorrect because it is a muscle of the neck that is responsible for rotating the head.

59. B: An anthrogenic gait is usually caused by osteoarthritis or rheumatoid arthritis and is often seen in older clients. Choice *A* refers to the causes of a Trendelenburg gait. Choice *C* refers to symptoms resulting in an antalgic gait, and the problems in Choice *D* result in an ataxic gait.

60. B: Proper hydration is important for athletes because it helps prevent cramping and muscle spasms. Choices *A*, *C*, and *D* are all benefits of hydration and of drinking water in particular, but these benefits are applicable to anybody, not just athletes.

61. C: Endangerment site refers to an area of the body where nerves and blood vessels are close to the surface and are not protected well. Choice *A*, areas of edema, is incorrect because these are areas where swelling is present. Choice *B*, local contraindication, is incorrect because that is a complication causing a specific area of the body to be painful, tender, or easily infected. As a result, massage therapists must modify a session to avoid that area. Choice *D*, trauma site, is incorrect because that is an area where an injury has occurred.

62. C: Traction is a technique used to elongate joints. It is most often done by a chiropractor but can be used during a massage as well. Stretching, Choice *A*, is a key part of any treatment and is used to relax and warm up muscles before treatment. Choice *B*, trigger point therapy, refers to a modality that stimulates a brain response to sensory input from an old injury. Joint mobilization, Choice *D*, is the physical manipulation of the joint by the therapist.

63. C: Thai massage, also called Thai yoga massage, incorporates assisted yoga positions into the massage session. Choices *A*, *B*, and *D* are all different massage modalities. Swedish massage is primarily a relaxing modality that uses light pressure and flowing movements. Sports massage is used for athletes either before or after competition. Prenatal massage focuses on expectant mothers and helps to relive conditions such as pregnancy-induced edema and sciatica.

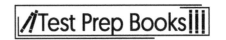

64. A: Pitted edema can be an indication of cardiovascular or kidney dysfunction. Contusions and hematomas, Choice *B*, are caused by injuries to small blood vessels and are usually visible on the surface of the skin or just beneath it. Choice *C*, varicose veins, are a visible spidering effect usually in the legs. Massaging a client with varicose veins can sometimes result in an embolism, Choice *D*.

65. C: ROM stands for the range of motion of a joint. It is usually measured in degrees. Choices *A*, *B*, and *D* are made-up answers.

66. B: Muscle spindles are proprioceptors that detect the magnitude and rate of muscle tension. Choice *A*, tropomyosin, is incorrect because tropomyosin is a protein that is a component of actin filaments. It is important in regulating muscle function. Choice *C*, sarcoplasm, is incorrect because that is the cytoplasm of muscle fiber. Choice *D*, myocytes, is incorrect because a myocyte is a muscle cell.

67. C: Obturator is the correct answer because the obturator foramen is located in the pelvis and allows nerves and blood vessels to pass from the abdomen into the legs. Choice *A*, ethmoid, is incorrect because the ethmoid foramen is located in the ethmoid bone of the skull. Choice *B*, lacerum, is incorrect because the lacerum foramen is on the temporal bone of the skull. Choice *D*, intervertebral, is incorrect because the intervertebral foramen is located in each vertebra and allows the nerve roots to exit the spinal column.

68. B: A dual relationship refers to situations in which the client is also a friend, relative, or business associate of the therapist. Therapists may provide a listening ear or be a comforting confidante to their clients fairly regularly during a therapy session, as in Choice *A*, but this is not the nature of a dual relationship. Similarly, Choices *C* and *D* may be true, but they are not representative of dual relationships

69. A: Palpation refers to the use of touch to identify specific muscles or anatomical structures, such as finding a particular vertebra along the spine. Choices *B*, *C*, and *D* refer to petrissage, effleurage, and tapotement, respectively, which are all different massage techniques.

70. D: The health history form does not include any preferences as to massage techniques or modalities. The health history form does, however, include all of the information listed in Choices *A*, *B*, and *C*, making Choice *D* the correct answer.

71. D: Boils is the correct answer because a boil is a pus-filled bump under the skin that most commonly develops from a Staphylococcus aureus infection. Choice *A*, herpes, is incorrect because that is the illness from a herpes simplex virus. Choice *B*, shingles, is incorrect because shingles is an issue that arises from the reactivation of the chickenpox virus. Choice *C*, plantar warts, is incorrect because these are rough growths on the feet that occur due to a human papillomavirus infection.

72. B: If a therapist has a conflicting opinion about the best treatment plan for a client, they should explain the benefits of the alternate approach and suggest the client do additional research. The therapist should never badmouth or gossip about other medical professionals, making Choices *A*, *C*, and *D* incorrect.

73. C: "Hair regrowing after being pulled out" is not a mechanism for maintaining homeostasis. Homeostasis is the process of the body maintaining balance in all of its systems, regulating temperature, levels of nutrients, blood pressure, and much more. Hair growth is not necessary for maintaining balance in any of the body's systems. Choice *A*, parathyroid releasing hormones when calcium levels are

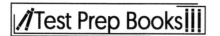

too low, is incorrect because that is a form of homeostatic regulation. Calcium levels that are too low or too high are dangerous to one's health, so proper levels must be regulated for homeostasis. Choice *B*, shivering in cold weather, is incorrect because shivering occurs to maintain body temperature when it drops to potentially dangerous levels. Choice *D*, sweat glands producing sweat when exposed to heat, is incorrect because sweat production is a homeostatic regulation that occurs when one is overheating. Sweat cools the body down to safe temperatures.

74. C: Endocrine is the correct answer because the pituitary gland, along with the adrenal glands, pancreas, and other glands, produce hormones to send signals throughout the body and make up the endocrine system. Choice *A*, circulatory, is incorrect because the circulatory system is composed of the heart and blood vessels and is designed to circulate blood. Choice *B*, nervous, is incorrect because the nervous system is made of the brain, spinal cord, and various neurons to transmit electrical signals throughout the body. Choice *D*, integumentary, is incorrect because the integumentary system is composed of the skin and acts as a physical barrier to protect the body.

75. A: The muscle energy technique is tailored to athletes to help optimize performance and facilitate post-event recovery. These techniques are not often appropriate with more fragile clients, such as those noted in Choices *B, C,* and *D*. Other techniques and considerations must be taken into account when working with these client groups.

76. C: The primary benefit and guiding principle in massage therapy is increasing the blood flow in the body. While Choices *A, B,* and *D* can be benefits of massage therapy, good blood and lymphatic flow are keys to whole-body healing and wellness, making Choice *C* the correct answer.

77. C: To maintain good body mechanics and avoid stress and strain on the therapist's body, the therapist should practice good posture, correct hand and arm techniques, and keep the massage table at an appropriate height, Choices *A, B,* and *D*. The therapist should maintain physical contact with the client as opposed to taking breaks during the sessions, making Choice *C* the correct answer.

78. A: The client's dietary restrictions are not required information for oncology massage. Choices *B, C,* and *D*, however, are important for the therapist to know.

79. A: Lordosis refers to an anterior tilt in the client's pelvis, commonly known as swayback. Choice *B* refers to a dowager's hump, while Choice *C* refers to scoliosis. Choice *D* describes a bridge, which is an exercise that is helpful in treating lordosis.

80. D: Craniosacral therapy is a form of bodywork involving the manipulation of joints in conjunction with the subtle, rhythmic movements of living tissue. Choice *A* is the definition of physiology, Choice *B* refers to effleurage, and Choice *C* refers to chair massage.

81. B: A therapist should always be wholly focused on a client during a massage therapy session. Stopping the session to take a phone call, while not an ethics violation as in Choice *A*, is a service violation and could result in a reprimand by their boss. The action does not constitute a violation of provider-patient confidentiality or a HIPAA violation, Choices *C* and *D*, unless the therapist discusses the patient with an outside party during the phone call.

82. C: Oxytocin is referred to as the "love hormone," as it is stimulated by touch and helps people bond with each other. Serotonin and dopamine, Choices *A* and *B*, are the other two neurotransmitters that

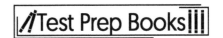

can have positive effects on the body. Cortisol, Choice *D*, is a hormone that can cause muscles to become tight and painful.

83. D: "The thumb is on the lateral side of the hand" is correct because in anatomical position, a person is standing upright with their thumbs facing outward on the lateral side of the hand. Choice *A*, the palms are facing backwards, is incorrect because in anatomical position, the palms face forward. Choice *B*, the body is lying down with the face up, is incorrect because the body is standing upright in anatomical position. Choice *C*, feet are flat and directed to the sides, is incorrect because in anatomical position, the feet are flat and directed forward.

84. B: Drop foot can be an indication of larger neurological and/or muscular issues. A hemiplegic gait results from the condition in Choice *A*. Choice *C* causes muscle contracture, while Choice *D* results in a scissors gait.

85. B: Information sent in the body of an email, as opposed to a password-protected attachment, is not secure and is susceptible to hacking. Client notes and records should never be sent this way. Choice *A* is incorrect if the client has signed the proper release forms; however, even if the client did sign release forms, client information should not be sent via the body of an email. Choice *C* is incorrect; medical professionals can share client records as necessary so long as the proper release forms have been signed. The amount of information included in SOAP notes varies from therapist to therapist and from practice to practice, making Choice *D* too vague. However, regardless of the level of detail, SOAP notes should never be sent in the body of an email.

86. B: Adjustments are typically done by chiropractors who are specifically trained in this type of joint manipulation. Aromatherapy, Choice *A*, refers to working with scents for specific purposes, such as alleviating anxiety. A reflexologist, Choice *C*, works with massaging specific areas of the feet to treat other parts of the body. Choice *D*, an esthetician, works primarily on improving a client's skin.

87. D: Ischial tuberosity is the correct answer because it is the rounded extended portion of the ischium that makes up the base of the pelvis. Choice *A*, deltoid tuberosity, is incorrect because that is a rough surface on the side of the humerus. Choice *B*, greater trochanter, is incorrect because that is a bony knob at the top of the femur that has an effect on the mechanical stress of the hip. Choice *C*, calcaneum, is incorrect because the calcaneum is the bone that forms the heel, which plays a role in stability and bearing weight.

88. C: Contraindications refer to medical issues that would preclude a client from receiving a massage, such as if a client is sick with the flu or has an open wound on the massage area. Choices *A*, *B*, and *D* are incorrect.

89. C: The scalene muscles are located in the neck. The purpose of the anterior scalene is to elevate the first rib to aid in respiration. Choice *A*, abdomen, is incorrect because the abdomen contains muscles such as the obliques, pyramidalis, and abdominis. Choice *B*, head, is incorrect because it contains muscles such as the masseter, temporalis, frontalis, and more, but not the scalene muscle. Choice *D*, back, is incorrect because it contains the latissimus dorsi, trapezius, rhomboids, and levator scapulae.

90. A: Cross-fiber friction refers to the deep-tissue massage technique of rubbing the muscle fibers perpendicular to the grain. Choice *B* refers to the incorrect direction (along the grain rather than perpendicular to it). Choices *C* and *D* refer to lighter, more superficial techniques.

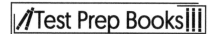
91. B: An insurance claim is used to bill the client's insurance for services provided. It usually includes the services that were provided, the dates, and the charges for those services. It is the first step is receiving reimbursement from the insurance company. Choices *A, C,* and *D* are incorrect.

92. C: Countertransference is when the therapist develops feelings for a client, whether romantic or platonic, outside of the professional relationship. While this is a somewhat common occurrence, acting on those feelings causes problems that can be damaging to both parties involved. Choice *D* refers to transference. Choices *A* and *B* are common situations in the therapist-client relationship, but do not relate to countertransference.

93. A: Tapotement is a percussive massage technique that consists of quick, well-aimed strokes. Choices *B, C,* and *D* all refer to other types of massage strokes. Effleurage is a gliding stroke with constant pressure. Petrissage is a kneading stroke used in deep-tissue work, and touch refers to static contact between the therapist and the client

94. A: HIPAA regulations indicate that physical patient records must be stored in a locked location. The rules do not specify that the room itself must be locked, Choice *B.* Under HIPAA regulations, a therapist who works in an office where medical records are transmitted to third parties, such as a chiropractor or physical therapist billing insurance companies for payment, is bound by HIPAA guidelines, making Choice *C* incorrect. Storing the records away from prying eyes is not sufficient if the records are not locked, as in Choice *D.*

95. A: Edema is the correct answer because it occurs when the interstitial space of tissues fills with fluid due to capillaries leaking. Choice *B,* allergies, is incorrect because allergies are an immune response, triggered by a substance, that can be damaging. Choice *C,* lymphoma, is incorrect because lymphoma is a cancer of the lymphatic system. Choice *D,* cellulitis, is incorrect because that is a bacterial infection that occurs under the skin.

96. D: Therapists who do not specialize can develop a broad, but limited, range of knowledge about a wide variety of treatment options. When a therapist specializes in a particular type of therapy, they are able to target a specific demographic of clients as in Choice *A,* such as pregnant women or competitive athletes. The therapist can also develop specific skills and knowledge involved in performing that particular style of therapy, Choice *B,* and they can build a private practice focusing specifically on that clientele, Choice *C.*

97. C: Cold therapy helps to control initial pain and reduce swelling. Choices *A, B,* and *D* all refer to the use of heat therapy in massage.

98. A: The phrase "scope of practice" refers to what a professional is and is not allowed to do within a work setting. While it may include references to office or practice policies or what services the practice offers, Choices *B, C,* and *D* are not the specific definition of the phrase.

99. C: Kyphosis is a forward protrusion of the head and neck, usually resulting from spending too much time hunched over a computer or desk. While Choices *A, B,* and *D* can certainly cause pain and injury, these are activities are not specific causes of kyphosis.

100. A: Cervical is the correct answer because the cervical region of the spinal column is above the lumbar and thoracic regions. In medical terminology, "superior" means above and "inferior" means below. Choice *B,* sacral, is incorrect because it is not a portion of the spinal column. The sacral region

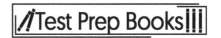

refers to the area of the body where the sacrum bone is, which is inferior to the lumbar region. Choice *C*, lumbar, is incorrect because it is the most inferior region of the spinal column. Choice *D*, thoracic, is incorrect because it is inferior to the cervical region.

Practice Test #4

1. Which statement about white blood cells is true?
   a. B cells are responsible for antibody production.
   b. White blood cells are made in the white/yellow cartilage before they enter the bloodstream.
   c. Platelets, a special class of white blood cell, function to clot blood and stop bleeding.
   d. The majority of white blood cells only activate during the age of puberty, which explains why children and the elderly are particularly susceptible to disease.

2. How do muscle fibers shorten during contraction?
   a. The actin filaments attach to the myosin, forming cross-bridges, and pull the fibers closer together.
   b. Calcium enters the sarcoplasmic reticulum, initiating an action potential.
   c. Myosin cross-bridges attach, rotate, and detach from actin filaments causing the ends of the sarcomere to be pulled closer together.
   d. The t-tubule system allows the fibers to physically shorten during contraction.

3. Is massage ever appropriate for a client with an autoimmune disease?
   a. No
   b. Yes, always
   c. Yes, but only during a flare-up
   d. Yes, but only during remission

4. Which branch of the nervous system does massage stimulate?
   a. The parasympathetic nervous system, which is part of the autonomic nervous system
   b. The sympathetic nervous system, which controls the fight-or-flight response
   c. The limbic system
   d. The central nervous system

5. Which of these conditions contraindicate massage?
   > I. Bruising
   > II. Edema
   > III. Pitted edema

   a. Choice I
   b. Choice III
   c. Choice II
   d. Choices I and III

6. As a massage therapist, following ethical guidelines is essential to one's success. Which of the following organizations lists the guidelines that should be followed?
   a. AMTA
   b. AARP
   c. NCBTMB
   d. A & C

7. When caring for fingernails, a therapist should do which of the following?
   a. Be extremely careful to groom hangnails and avoid nail polish
   b. Make sure the nails are pleasing to the eye; they are a valuable advertisement
   c. Get weekly manicures
   d. Trim them at least every two days

8. Which locations in the digestive system are sites of chemical digestion?
   I. Mouth
   II. Stomach
   III. Small Intestine

   a. II only
   b. III only
   c. II and III only
   d. I, II, and III

9. Which of the following is not considered to be a primary function of the proprioceptive system?
   a. Provide awareness of position and kinesthesia within the surroundings
   b. Produce coordinated reflexes to maintain muscle tone and balance
   c. Provide peripheral feedback information to the central nervous system to help modify movements and motor response
   d. Provide cushioning to joints during impact

10. Which of the following is an endangerment site?
    a. The Posterior Popliteal Notch
    b. The Occiput
    c. The Anterior Triangle of the Neck
    d. The Inguinal Canal

11. When it comes to maintaining personal boundaries with a client, which of the following is true?
    a. It is fine to date a client as long as the attraction and feelings are mutual.
    b. If a client shares personal problems with the therapist, then it is fine for the therapist to share their personal problems with the client.
    c. If working within one's home, the designated massage room can be a spare bedroom.
    d. Therapists must not burden clients with their own personal problems.

12. When draping a client, the therapist should do which of the following?
    a. Work through the sheet, keeping the client's body covered at all times
    b. Uncover the area being worked on, taking care to create a clear boundary
    c. Only drape the client if requested to do so
    d. Ask the client whether they prefer to be draped

13. What effect does massage have on serotonin levels?
    a. Massage causes serotonin to bond with lactic acid
    b. Massage prevents the body from processing serotonin
    c. Massage increases serotonin levels in both the client and the therapist
    d. Massage has no impact on serotonin

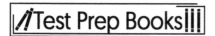

14. A client tells his therapist that he is interested in cupping. The therapist is not trained in that modality, but he or she believes it could be useful for this particular client's condition. What should the therapist do?

    a. Invest in the proper supplies and try cupping with the client. The customer is always right.

    b. Discourage the client from seeking cupping. It might be helpful, but it is more important to retain business.

    c. Refer the client to another therapist trained in this modality.

    d. Try cupping with the client, using supplies already on hand.

15. Why do arteries have valves?

    a. They have valves to maintain high blood pressure so that capillaries diffuse nutrients properly.

    b. Their valves are designed to prevent backflow due to their low blood pressure.

    c. The valves have no known purpose and thus appear to be unnecessary.

    d. They do not have valves, but veins do.

16. Which of the following correctly explains the order of how muscle spindles sense the rate and magnitude of increasing muscle tension as the muscle lengthens?

    a. The muscle spindle is stretched, sensory neurons in the spindle are activated, an impulse is sent to the spinal cord, motor neurons that innervate extrafusal fibers are signaled to relax

    b. The muscle spindle is stretched, motor neurons in the spindle are activated, an impulse is sent to the spinal cord, sensory neurons that innervate extrafusal fibers are signaled to relax

    c. Sensory neurons in the spindle are activated, the muscle spindle is stretched, an impulse is sent to the spinal cord, motor neurons that innervate extrafusal fibers are signaled to relax

    d. The muscle spindle is stretched, sensory neurons in the spindle are activated, an impulse is sent to the spinal cord, sensory neurons that innervate intrafusal fibers are signaled to relax

17. If a therapist violates one or more of the codes of ethics, it is possible, depending on the severity of the violation, for which of the following to occur?

    a. The therapist receives a verbal warning from management.

    b. The therapist gets fired.

    c. The therapist gets arrested.

    d. All of the above

18. What does SOAP stand for?

    a. Subject, Observations, Affect, Purpose

    b. Subjective, Objective, Assessment, Plan

    c. Supine, Opposition, Abductor, Prone

    d. Subjective, Observation, Allocate, Plan

19. Is massage indicated for clients experiencing muscle spasm due to injury?

    a. Yes, massage should be used to relax injured muscles, completely relieving spasms as soon as possible.

    b. Yes, but the therapist should be careful not to relieve the spasm entirely.

    c. No, massage should never be performed on clients with muscle spasms.

    d. Yes, but massage should be performed only distal to the site of the injury.

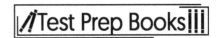

20. Which of these acronyms stands for the law protecting the privacy of medical patients, including massage clients?
    a. SOAP
    b. HIPAA
    c. MET
    d. FHP

21. Which of the following is true regarding tipping?
    a. It is considered unethical. A therapist should dismiss clients who offer them tips.
    b. It is a necessary percentage of any LMT's income. Calculate all wages + 20% in tips when considering a new job.
    c. It is more common in spas and hotels than medical clinics.
    d. It is an accepted practice, but therapists should refuse them if trying to be professional.

22. If the pressure in the pulmonary artery is increased above normal, which chamber of the heart will be affected first?
    a. The right atrium
    b. The left atrium
    c. The right ventricle
    d. The left ventricle

23. After assessing a client's passive range of motion in the knee, the therapist determines there is limitation in flexion. Which of the following list of structures may be responsible for the restricted range of motion?
    a. Quadriceps, ligaments, knee joint capsule, fascia
    b. Hamstrings, ligaments, knee joint capsule, fascia
    c. Gastrocnemius, ligaments, knee joint capsule, fascia
    d. Ligaments, knee joint capsule, fascia

24. Which of the following is considered a violation of the code of ethics?
    a. Talking poorly about a client with another therapist in a public area where that client can hear.
    b. Having to cut a client's time short a few minutes because he or she was late and another client is scheduled immediately afterward.
    c. Privately discussing a client's musculoskeletal issue with another therapist to receive advice on how to proceed with the treatment.
    d. Terminating a massage therapy session immediately upon the client making an inappropriate advance to the therapist.

25. How does massage impact blood flow?
    a. Massage has no impact on blood flow
    b. Massage increases blood flow only to the areas treated
    c. Massage increases the flow of blood and lymph throughout the body
    d. Massage decreases blood flow to the areas treated

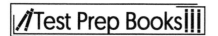

26. A therapist has spent her career working in hospitals and medical facilities. She gets a new job at a 5-star hotel that has very specific draping requirements. What should she do?
    a. On her first day, explain to the first client that she is still in training and learn on her first client
    b. Bring her own sheets to the new job
    c. Explain to her new employer that she already knows how to drape
    d. Practice draping at home on a friend or family member

27. A client with fibromyalgia suffers from which of the following?
    a. Chronic pain
    b. Acute pain
    c. Hypertonic IT bands
    d. Poor circulation

28. During an intake, a client mentions that she has been taking blood thinners. This may be indicative of which of the following?
    a. The client is hypertensive.
    b. The client has recently given birth.
    c. The client is at high risk for clotting.
    d. The client is both hypertensive and at high risk for clotting.

29. What is the purpose of sodium bicarbonate when released into the lumen of the small intestine?
    a. It works to chemically digest fats in the chyme.
    b. It decreases the pH of the chyme so as to prevent harm to the intestine.
    c. It works to chemically digest proteins in the chyme.
    d. It increases the pH of the chyme so as to prevent harm to the intestine.

30. Which of the following lists of joint types is in the correct order for increasing amounts of permitted motion (least mobile to most mobile)?
    a. Hinge, condyloid, saddle
    b. Saddle, hinge, condyloid
    c. Saddle, condyloid, hinge
    d. Hinge, saddle, condyloid

31. What is the psychological term used to describe the therapeutic relationship between the therapist and the client?
    a. Power play
    b. Power differential
    c. Power couple
    d. Power relationship

32. Why is table height important?
    I. Choosing the proper table height allows the therapist to use appropriate body mechanics and avoid injury.
    II. A higher table is better for sports massage, while a lower table is better for prenatal work.
    III. Table height impacts the amount of pressure the therapist can apply. The lower the table, the more pressure is possible.

    a. I, II, III
    b. II, III
    c. I only
    d. I, III

33. Which of the following is/are true regarding muscles that are hypertonic?
    I. They suffer from poor circulation.
    II. They may be constricted by the formation of scar tissue.
    III. They can be most effectively treated with tapotement.

    a. I
    b. II
    c. III
    d. I and II

34. Is massage indicated for clients in high-stress jobs?
    a. No, they don't have the time for massage
    b. Yes, massage can help relieve stress
    c. Yes, massage can take the place of talk therapy
    d. No, massage increases stress levels in some clients

35. Which of the following is an example of a dual relationship?
    a. Massaging one's sibling
    b. Going to an art exhibit with a client (not as a date)
    c. Bartering with a client for a haircut and color
    d. All of the above

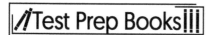

36. Which of the following is the correct sequence of the 3 primary body planes as numbered 1, 2, and 3 in the following image?

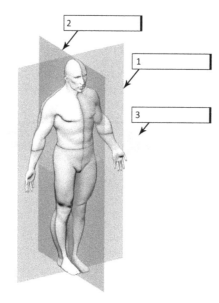

a. Plane 1 is coronal, plane 2 is sagittal, and plane 3 is transverse.
b. Plane 1 is sagittal, plane 2 is coronal, and plane 3 is medial.
c. Plane 1 is coronal, plane 2 is sagittal, and plane 3 is medial.
d. Plane 1 is sagittal, plane 2 is coronal, and plane 3 is transverse.

37. Which of the following is NOT a component of a sarcomere?
a. Actin
b. D-line
c. A-Band
d. I-Band

38. Muscle energy technique can cause changes in which of the following?
a. Proprioception
b. Digestion
c. Lymphatic circulation
d. Parasympathetic state

39. What is the difference between acute and chronic pain?
a. Acute pain is caused by impact; chronic pain is caused by poor body mechanics
b. Acute pain is caused by injury; chronic pain lasts longer than 6 weeks
c. Acute pain is caused by injury; chronic pain is caused by poor nutrition
d. Acute pain lasts for less than a week; chronic pain never heals

40. How likely is it that an employer will require a practical interview?
    a. Very unlikely. Practicals are going out of style.
    b. Very likely. In fact, the therapist should be wary of any interviews that do away with the practical component.
    c. Very unlikely. It is awkward to see a potential employer naked.
    d. Very likely. It is customary for the therapist to work on an easily accessible part of the body, like the hands or feet.

41. Is it ever appropriate to massage a client who is paraplegic and wheelchair-bound?
    a. Yes, but massage should only be performed if he or she is under the age of 60.
    b. Yes, but work on an atrophied limb is contraindicated.
    c. Yes, working on atrophied limbs can improve blood and lymph flow throughout the body.
    d. No, it is dangerous to work on a wheelchair-bound client.

42. Which of the client's bodily fluids should the therapist avoid, according to standard precautions?
    a. Blood and pus only. All other fluids are safe as long as the therapist has no open wounds and washes their hands immediately.
    b. All bodily fluids, including but not limited to blood, sweat, tears, semen, vaginal secretions, mucus, saliva, and pus.
    c. Most bodily fluids, including blood, sweat, semen, vaginal secretions, mucus, saliva, and pus.
    d. Most bodily fluids, but not including sweat.

43. Which of the following is NOT a major function of the respiratory system in humans?
    a. It provides a large surface area for gas exchange of oxygen and carbon dioxide.
    b. It helps regulate the blood's pH.
    c. It helps cushion the heart against jarring motions.
    d. It is responsible for vocalization.

44. Which of the following correctly lists the structures of a muscle from largest to smallest?
    a. Fasciculus, muscle fiber, actin, myofibril
    b. Muscle fiber, fasciculus, myofibril, actin
    c. Sarcomere, fasciculus, myofibril, myosin
    d. Muscle fiber, myofibril, sarcomere, actin

45. Which of these can cause painful muscle cramps and spasms?
    I. Sodium imbalance
    II. Calcium imbalance
    III. Potassium imbalance

    a. I
    b. II
    c. III
    d. I, II, and III

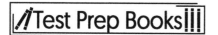

46. Why is resting position important?
    a. So the client has the opportunity to fall asleep
    b. So the client and therapist can relax and communicate via touch
    c. So the therapist gets a break from their busy day
    d. So the client's heart rate can slow down

47. When a client develops an attachment to a therapist because the client feels that the therapist is the only one that listens to all of their personal problems as well as fixing muscular ones, this is an example of which of the following?
    a. Countertransference
    b. Transference
    c. Bartering
    d. Dating

48. What is acupuncture?
    a. A recently developed style of bodywork that involves placing needles in tight muscles to release physical tension.
    b. An ancient form of medicine developed in India.
    c. An ancient holistic modality that involves placing needles at specific points in the body.
    d. A recently developed Eastern modality intended to alleviate anxiety by releasing endorphins.

49. What should the therapist do if a client makes an overt sexual advance toward a therapist during a session?
    a. Try to change the subject
    b. Politely ask the client to stop
    c. Ignore the advance
    d. Terminate the session immediately and report the incident to management and/or security

50. Which of the following is NOT a function of the forebrain?
    a. To regulate blood pressure and heart rate
    b. To perceive and interpret emotional responses like fear and anger
    c. To perceive and interpret visual input from the eyes
    d. To integrate voluntary movement

51. Myosin cross-bridges attach to the actin filament when the sarcoplasmic reticulum is stimulated to release which of the following?
    a. Calcium ions
    b. Acetylcholine
    c. Troponin
    d. Adenosine triphosphate (ATP)

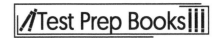

52. What does "proximal/distal/proximal" refer to?
    a. When working on a limb, the therapist should start as far away from the heart as possible and work back toward the torso.
    b. When working on the back, the therapist should start with broad, general strokes and gradually become more specific.
    c. When working on a limb, the therapist should use progressively deeper pressure, ending with the firmest touch of all.
    d. When working on a limb, the therapist should address the entire limb, starting and ending the session at the shoulder or the hip. This remains true even if the site of pain is at the distal end of the limb.

53. A client with kyphotic posture would display which of the following?
    a. A swayback
    b. Medially rotated shoulders, with the head protruding past the mid-sagittal line
    c. Hyperextension of the knees
    d. Drop foot

54. Which of the following statements about regulations is true?
    a. Every state has licensing laws.
    b. Every state has the same regulations regarding massage therapy.
    c. It is necessary to attend an accredited massage school to get a license.
    d. A therapist's individual state license is valid in other states.

55. A therapist is trained in aromatherapy and keeps essential oils on hand for use during treatment. A new client complains of intense anxiety. The therapist believes aromatherapy can help. What is the best course of action?
    a. Use the proper essential oils during massage without mentioning it to the client. Asking too many questions will just make the client more anxious.
    b. Explain the history of aromatherapy and the client's different options. The client can only make an informed decision if they understand every detail of the recommended treatment.
    c. Offer the client one or two options after asking about any allergies they have. Then just go with whichever one you feel is best.
    d. Prescribe lavender. It will alleviate the client's symptoms.

56. Which of the following statements is FALSE?
    a. Painkillers have short-term benefits but can cause health problems in the long term.
    b. Painkillers can damage the stomach, but there is no risk of addiction.
    c. Some painkillers are available over the counter; others must be prescribed by a doctor.
    d. Painkillers classified as opioids are derived from opium.

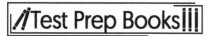

57. The function of synergists can best be described as which of the following?
    I. They assist primary movers in completing the specific movement
    II. They stabilize the point of origin and provide extra pull near the insertion
    III. They help prevent unwanted movement at a joint

    a. I, II
    b. I, III
    c. II, III
    d. All of the above

58. Which of the following types of joints are correctly matched with the anatomic joint example given?
    I. Cartilaginous: pubic symphysis
    II. Saddle: thumb carpal-metacarpal
    III. Plane: sutures in skull
    IV. Pivot: radial head on ulna

    a. Choices I, II, and III
    b. Choices I, II, and IV
    c. Choices I, III, and IV
    d. All are correct

59. Gait assessment can indicate which of the following?
    a. The presence of adhesions
    b. Inadequate hydration
    c. Muscle imbalance resulting from misaligned posture
    d. Factors that contraindicate massage

60. Overuse of heat therapy can result in which of the following?
    a. Overstimulation of the inflammatory response
    b. Third-degree burns
    c. Unnecessary pain
    d. All of the above

61. When might a therapist offer a chair massage?
    a. Chair massage is useful for prenatal work, especially during the third trimester. Many people have trouble lying down during this time, so sitting is a better option.
    b. Chair massage is a valuable way to promote massage therapy to the general public. Try setting up in an office or on a beach—the client doesn't need to disrobe, and passersby will want to learn more.
    c. Chair massage is only offered in medical settings like hospitals or nursing homes.
    d. Chair massage is most effective in the morning.

62. Bruegger's Relief Position is a self-care exercise that alleviates what condition?
    a. Kyphosis
    b. Lordosis
    c. Hypertonic IT bands
    d. Antalgic gait

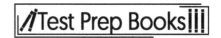

63. Which of the following is a type of energy work?
   a. Cryotherapy
   b. Reiki
   c. Aromatherapy
   d. Sports Massage (particularly pre-competition)

64. What makes bone resistant to shattering?
   a. The calcium salts deposited in the bone
   b. The collagen fibers
   c. The bone marrow and network of blood vessels
   d. The intricate balance of minerals and collagen fibers

65. Which of the following upper body movements take place in the sagittal plane?
       I. Elbow extension
       II. Wrist flexion
       III. Shoulder abduction
       IV. Neck left tilt

   a. I and IV
   b. I, III, IV
   c. I and II
   d. II and III

66. What does PROM stand for?
   a. Painful Range of Motion
   b. Pain-free Range of Motion
   c. Prone, Range of motion, Optimize, Manipulate
   d. Palpate Range of Motion

67. Which of the following is NOT part of a massage therapist's scope of practice?
   a. A therapist is able to diagnose a client's medical or musculoskeletal issues.
   b. A therapist can only practice modalities in which he or she is properly trained.
   c. A therapist assessing a client's conditions and notating anything unusual they find.
   d. A therapist must follow the guidelines set forth by their workplace regarding certain services that a massage therapist may or may not perform, such as body treatments.

68. What is a deductible?
   a. The amount of money an insured client is expected to pay for one office visit
   b. The amount the insurance company pays after receiving a claim
   c. The maximum amount of money an insurance plan will allow a patient to pay for care in a given year
   d. A set amount of money that the client must pay before their insurance begins to cover the costs of care

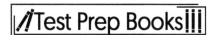

69. Which of the following statements is true regarding the first trimester of pregnancy?
    a. Massage is extremely dangerous during this time.
    b. There is no risk of morning sickness during this time.
    c. There is a high risk of miscarriage.
    d. The pubic symphysis always separates.

70. If a massage therapist suspects a client is intoxicated what should he or she do?
    a. Proceed with the session, using light touch only
    b. Consult his or supervisor because intoxication is an absolute contraindication
    c. Ask them if they have recently consumed alcohol
    d. Proceed with the session as he or she would otherwise

71. Using anatomical terms, what is the relationship of the sternum relative to the deltoid?
    a. Medial
    b. Lateral
    c. Superficial
    d. Posterior

72. What muscle is the primary antagonist in knee flexion?
    a. Hamstrings
    b. Quadriceps
    c. Gastrocnemius
    d. Tibialis anterior

73. During an intake, a client mentions that she regularly sees an acupuncturist who has prescribed her a regimen of herbs and supplements. What is the best course of action?
    a. Refuse treatment. Acupuncture and massage should not be combined.
    b. Ask what exactly she is taking, and research the effects of her prescriptions before performing massage.
    c. Proceed with the intake, but do not waste time asking more questions. Herbs are not as strong as prescription drugs.
    d. It depends on her reason for seeking treatment. If she has an acute muscle injury, the herbs will be flushed from her system due to immune response.

74. Does massage impact mental health?
    a. No, massage is only meant to heal sore muscles.
    b. No, massage therapists must keep clear boundaries.
    c. Yes, massage can directly improve a client's mental health.
    d. Yes, but indirectly: releasing muscle tension can improve a client's mood.

75. A weak or misfiring gluteus medius can result in which of the following gait deviations?
    a. Trendelenburg's gait
    b. Arthrogenic gait
    c. Ataxic gait
    d. Psoatic limp gait

76. Which of the following is NOT true about communication?
    a. Clients must communicate clearly with therapists.
    b. Therapists must communicate clearly with other therapists.
    c. Management doesn't have to communicate clearly with either clients or therapists.
    d. Therapists must communicate clearly with clients.

77. A regular client comes in for his session, obviously flushed and sweating. He sneezes repeatedly in the waiting room and mentions during the intake that he "really hopes this will make me feel better." What is the best course of action?
    a. Fire him as a client. It is unethical for him to expose you to illness.
    b. Go along with the session as if nothing were unusual. It would be rude to mention that he's obviously ill.
    c. Politely suggest that he come back another day because massage is contraindicated with a fever.
    d. Offer to do lymphatic drainage work, since it will stimulate blood flow and flush out his system.

78. What do nociceptors detect?
    a. Temperature
    b. Movement
    c. Pain
    d. Vibration

79. What is joint mobilization?
    a. The gentle movement of a client's joint by the therapist
    b. The movement of any joint in the body
    c. The firm movement of a client's joint by the therapist, stretching the tendons and ligaments to test their end feel
    d. An active movement of the client during a massage, against the therapist's resistance

80. Which of the following should ideally NOT be induced by massage?
    a. Cortisol release
    b. Flatulence
    c. Sleep
    d. A parasympathetic state

81. What are skeletal muscles?
    a. Muscles that attach to the skeleton
    b. Muscles that a person can move voluntarily
    c. Both A and B are correct
    d. All muscles are skeletal muscles

82. Which of the following bodywork techniques or modalities is used primarily to treat back and neck pain?
    a. Reflexology
    b. Tractioning
    c. Reiki
    d. Cryotherapy

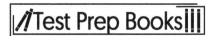
83. Are massage therapists held to HIPAA laws?
    a. Yes
    b. No
    c. Only if the place of business is considered a covered entity under HIPAA regulations
    d. Only if the place of business decides to follow HIPAA laws on its own

84. Is it appropriate to work on a client who took Advil twenty minutes prior to the massage?
    a. No, it isn't.
    b. Yes, it is.
    c. Effleurage is contraindicated, but deep tissue work is safe.
    d. It depends on the client's reason for taking Advil.

85. Which of the following is true regarding the connective tissue enclosing muscles and other organs?
    a. It is called fascia and can be released via myofascial stretching and skin rolling.
    b. It is called the protective sheath and can be released using Muscle Energy Technique.
    c. It is called the pericardium and can be released with transverse friction.
    d. It is called interstitial tissue and can be released with lymphatic drainage.

86. What does PRICE mean?
    a. Pain, Range of Motion, Instability, Clenching, Eversion
    b. Pressure, Release, Inversion, Cold, Elevation
    c. Pressure, Relaxation, Ice, Corrective posture, Exam
    d. Protection, Rest, Ice, Compression, Elevation

87. Where should sensitive information about clients be kept?
    a. In a folder on a desk
    b. In a locked file cabinet or on a password-protected computer
    c. In a drawer in the massage room
    d. At the reception area

88. How should the therapist breathe during a massage?
    a. It doesn't matter; the important thing is for the client to breathe deeply.
    b. The therapist should breathe silently, so as not to disturb the client.
    c. The therapist should breathe deeply. If the client hears this, it will inspire them to do the same.
    d. The therapist should breathe in through the nose for 6 counts and out through the mouth for 8 counts.

89. Which statement about Autonomic Nervous System drugs is correct?
    a. Anticholinergics stimulate muscle growth.
    b. Antiadrenergic drugs increase the fight-or-flight response and are used during heart attacks.
    c. Cholinergic drugs are sometimes called sympatholytic drugs.
    d. Adrenergic drugs can be used during medical crises.

90. Which of the following are principles of massage therapy?
    a. Increased circulation
    b. Stretching muscles
    c. Bridging the mind-body connection
    d. All of the above.

91. Positive rest position primarily targets which muscle group?
    a. Hamstrings
    b. Hip flexors
    c. Quadratus lumborum
    d. Erector spinae

92. Tapotement should be done in what way?
    a. Painful
    b. Invigorating
    c. Deep enough to bruise
    d. Light and feathery

93. What is a finger cot?
    a. A small cut near the cuticle
    b. A kind of liquid bandage
    c. A latex barrier used to cover a single finger
    d. A latex barrier taped to the client's skin

94. Which of the following is not technically considered a modality of massage therapy?
    a. Reflexology
    b. Deep Tissue
    c. Hot Stone
    d. Swedish

95. Wall angels can help with which of the following?
    a. Relieve pain in the rhomboids
    b. Correct medial rotation of the shoulders
    c. Stretch the pectoral muscles
    d. All of the above

96. What type of client should NOT receive a deep tissue massage?
    a. Someone who doesn't like pain
    b. Someone who has a lot of trigger points
    c. Someone who has high blood pressure or diabetes that is not regulated by medication
    d. Someone who isn't athletic

97. Which of the following are stroke techniques used in Swedish massage?
    a. Petrissage
    b. Effleurage
    c. Tapotement
    d. All of the above

98. What is the difference between a strain and a sprain?
    a. A strain involves a damaged muscle or tendon; a sprain involves a damaged ligament.
    b. A sprain is more serious than a strain.
    c. A strain can be classified as Grade I, Grade II, or Grade III.
    d. There is no difference; these words can be used interchangeably.

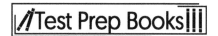

99. A weak gluteus medius and tight IT bands can result in which of the following conditions?
    a. Tension headaches
    b. Swayback
    c. Patellar instability
    d. TMJ

100. To what temperature should stones be heated for a hot stone massage?
    a. 80-100 degrees
    b. 120-150 degrees
    c. 70-90 degrees
    d. 180-200 degrees

Answer Explanations #4

1. A: When activated, B cells create antibodies against specific antigens. White blood cells are generated in red and yellow bone marrow, not cartilage. Platelets are not a type of white blood cell and are typically cell fragments produced by megakaryocytes. White blood cells are active throughout nearly all of one's life and have not been shown to specially activate or deactivate because of life events like puberty or menopause.

2. C: During muscle contractions, myosin cross-bridges attach via their globular heads to actin, then they swivel and detach from actin filaments, causing the ends of the sarcomere to be pulled closer together. Choice *A* is incorrect because it is essentially the opposite of this. Actin (the thin filament) does not attach to myosin (the thick filament). Choice *B* is incorrect because the action potential is initiated when calcium leaves—rather than enters—the sarcoplasmic reticulum. Choice *D* is wrong because fibers do not physically shorten. They slide past one another, shortening the distance between the origin and insertion of the muscle.

3. D: Yes, but only during remission. Massage can be extremely helpful for clients with autoimmune disorders, such as multiple sclerosis or lupus, as it helps the body heal from the stress and injury sustained during a flare-up. Massage is contraindicated during flare-ups of these conditions because it may increase inflammation and exacerbate symptoms.

4. A: The nervous system has many branches (broken down below). Massage stimulates the parasympathetic nervous system (or PSNS), which controls the body's rest-and-digest response.

> I. Central Nervous System
>
>> i. Brain
>>
>> ii. Spinal Cord
>
> II. Peripheral Nervous System (PNS)
>
>> i. Somatic Nerves: control voluntary actions, such as skeletal muscle movements
>>
>> ii. Autonomic Nervous System (ANS): controls involuntary actions, such as digestion and breathing
>>
>>> a. Sympathetic Nervous System: controls fight-or-flight response
>>>
>>> b. Parasympathetic Nervous System (PSNS): controls rest-and-digest response.

5. D: A bruise forms due to blood vessels breaking beneath the skin. Massaging a bruise can increase bleeding. While massage can actually be helpful in reducing edema (swelling), pitted edema (swollen tissue retains an indentation when pressed) can indicate cirrhosis of the liver, malfunctioning kidneys, or congestive heart failure. Bruising and pitted edema are both *local* contraindications rather than general ones, which means that therapists should simply avoid massaging the affected area. While it is not within a massage therapist's scope of practice to diagnose medical conditions, clients displaying symptoms of pitted edema should be encouraged to consult a physician.

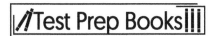

6. D: The AMTA and the NCBTMB are the largest and most popular professional associations in the massage therapy industry.

7. A: Be extremely careful to groom hangnails and avoid nail polish. Hangnails can be dangerous for the therapist and client alike, as they can easily break the skin. They can also be uncomfortable and are viewed as unprofessional in this field. Nail polish is unacceptable at work, as it harbors bacteria. It may be pleasing to the eye, but it increases the risk of contagion between client and therapist.

8. D: Mechanical digestion is physical digestion of food and tearing it into smaller pieces using force. This occurs in the stomach and mouth. Chemical digestion involves chemically changing the food and breaking it down into small organic compounds that can be utilized by the cell to build molecules. The salivary glands in the mouth secrete amylase that breaks down starch, which begins chemical digestion. The stomach contains enzymes such as pepsinogen/pepsin and gastric lipase, which chemically digest protein and fats, respectively. The small intestine continues to digest protein using the enzymes trypsin and chymotrypsin. It also digests fats with the help of bile from the liver and lipase from the pancreas. These organs act as exocrine glands because they secrete substances through a duct. Carbohydrates are digested in the small intestine with the help of pancreatic amylase, gut bacterial flora and fauna, and brush border enzymes like lactose. Brush border enzymes are contained in the towel-like microvilli in the small intestine that soak up nutrients.

9. D: Cartilage and synovial fluid are the primary sources of cushioning to joints during impact. The proprioceptive system is responsible for body awareness, coordinated reflexes for balance, and modifying movements based on neural feedback.

10. C: The Anterior Triangle of the Neck contains many delicate structures, including the jugular vein, the carotid artery, and the vagus nerve. The Popliteal Fossa (*not* referred to as a notch) is also an endangerment zone, as is the Inguinal Triangle. The Inguinal Canal is a structure that borders the Inguinal Triangle; in and of itself, it is not considered an endangerment site. The muscles surrounding the occiput can benefit from deep pressure, depending on the client's specific needs.

11. D: Therapists should not burden their clients with their personal problems. Clients often seek massage therapy to relax and escape the stress of their daily lives, and listening to a therapist's problems is not an ideal way to relax. While sometimes clients find it relaxing and therapeutic to discuss their own issues during a massage, good therapists listen and occasionally comment, rather than sharing their own stories.

12. B: Draping is required by law in the United States, helps to maintain client privacy, and sets professional boundaries. Areas of the body not being worked on should be draped. Female breast tissue and genitals must always remain covered. Sheets used for draping should not be translucent.

13. C: Massage increases serotonin levels in both the client and the therapist. Production and reuptake of serotonin are stimulated by any skin-to-skin contact. (This is also true for dopamine and oxytocin.) Because both the client and therapist are experiencing this kind of touch during a treatment, serotonin levels will increase in both people. Note that the serotonin levels of the client are more drastically affected than those of the therapist. By increasing levels of these three neurotransmitters, massage promotes a sense of happiness and well-being.

14. C: Refer the client to another therapist who is trained in this modality. A therapist's first responsibility is to facilitate the client's healing process. If another provider can offer more effective

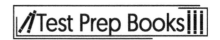

treatment, the therapist should refer the client out. A therapist should never offer a service in which s/he is not sufficiently trained.

15. D: Veins have valves, but arteries do not. Valves in veins are designed to prevent backflow, since they are the furthest blood vessels from the pumping action of the heart and steadily increase in volume (which decreases the available pressure). Capillaries diffuse nutrients properly because of their thin walls and high surface area and are not particularly dependent on positive pressure.

16. A: Muscle spindles are made of intrafusal muscle fibers, running parallel to the direction of the extrafusal fibers. When a muscle is stretched, the embedded spindles are also stretched, activating sensory neurons in the spindles. This activation sends an impulse to the spinal cord, where the sensory neurons synapse with motor neurons. These motor neurons exit the spinal cord and travel back towards the limb, where they innervate the extrafusal fibers, which receive the message to relax.

17. D: Working within the code of ethics as set forth by professional associations or one's workplace is a great way to avoid any disciplinary issues. However, if a therapist violates the code of ethics, there are numerous disciplinary options, depending on the severity of the violation. A therapist can receive anything from a verbal warning for a minor infraction, to job termination or even arrest for something such as a sexual misconduct violation.

18. B: Subjective, Objective, Assessment, Plan. Subjective notes include anything the client says to the therapist. Objective notes are the therapist's specific, scientific findings. Assessment includes the therapist's clinical assessment of the client's condition (not a diagnosis) and a description of what they did during today's treatment. The plan describes any homework assigned to the client and the intended course of action going forward. For example:

> S: Client complains of shoulder pain, made worse when she holds her 3-month-old daughter.

> O: Decreased R shoulder flexion.

> A: Myofascial adhesions and hypertonicity in R biceps brachii, R anterior deltoid, and R brachialis. Applied myofascial release to the shoulder girdle, including the muscles listed above, R scalenes, and R SITS muscles.

> P: Recommended door frame stretches twice daily. Client will return in one week. If adhesions are still present, the treatment will include deep cross-fiber friction techniques. If adhesions have healed by the time of the session, we will re-assess.

19. B: Yes, but the therapist should be careful not to relieve the spasm entirely. Muscle spasms are painful, and many people seek massage to alleviate them. However, they almost always serve a very specific function. Muscles go into spasm in order to protect from further injury—they might be protecting a damaged joint capsule or holding an intervertebral disc in place to prevent further herniation. The therapist should do their best to relieve some pain, but be careful not to cause the very damage the spasm is preventing.

20. B: HIPAA stands for the Health Insurance Portability and Accountability Act. It mandates that healthcare professionals, including massage therapists, maintain patient confidentiality, meaning that it is not appropriate to disclose a client's information, including their name, health conditions, and any other personal details, to a third party.

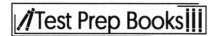
SOAP (subjective, objective, action, plan) notes are used to record the information that a client shares during verbal intake, the information that a therapist observes about a client's tissues during visual and palpation assessment, the techniques used to treat the client during the massage session, and the treatment plan devised for future sessions.

MET, or Muscle Energy Technique, is a kind of stretching that expands a client's proprioception. MET is commonly used during sports massage to alleviate muscle spasm or strain.

Forward head posture (FHP), in which the neck and head protrude past the vertical reference line, is often caused by long hours spent hunched over a computer or textbook.

21. C: It is more common in spas and hotels than medical clinics. Tips are always nice, but a therapist should never depend on them for income. Clients are changeable—sometimes the same person will tip generously on one occasion, and not at all on another. Clients generally assume that tips are inappropriate in medical settings. Some doctors agree and discourage clinical LMTs from accepting gratuity.

22. C: The blood leaves the right ventricle through a semi-lunar valve and goes through the pulmonary artery to the lungs. Any increase in pressure in the artery will eventually affect the contractibility of the right ventricle. Blood enters the right atrium from the superior and inferior venae cava veins, and blood leaves the right atrium through the tricuspid valve to the right ventricle. Blood enters the left atrium from the pulmonary veins carrying oxygenated blood from the lungs. Blood flows from the left atrium to the left ventricle through the mitral valve and leaves the left ventricle through a semi-lunar valve to enter the aorta.

23. D: Passive range of motion assesses the non-contractile joint structures, such as ligaments, capsules, and fascia. Active range of motion would also assess the contractile elements, such as muscles and tendons, in addition to the non-contractile elements. Therefore, the specific muscles involved in knee flexion were not applicable to this question.

24. A: Creating a positive experience for the client goes beyond just the massage session itself. Making a client feel safe and emotionally secure is also part of the process. If clients hear therapists speak poorly of them, it will not only ruin the overall experience, but it also will deeply hurt them. This is a betrayal of trust.

25. C: Massage increases the flow of blood and lymph throughout the body. Massage has a strong positive effect on circulation. This increases the volume of blood and lymph in the entire circulatory system. The therapist should bear this in mind, especially when working with hypertensive clients who already have unnecessary stress on their cardiovascular system.

26. D: Practice draping at home on a friend or family member. Different draping techniques are necessary in different settings, and, above all, a therapist should follow the professional standards set forth by the state and employer. Clients have extremely varied expectations about modesty depending on the setting. Whatever the setting, it is the therapist's responsibility to meet the client's expectations.

27. A: Chronic pain differs from acute pain in its duration. While acute pain comes on suddenly, often as a result of injury and tends to be sharp, chronic pain can linger after an injury has healed or result from underlying health conditions. Fibromyalgia is a condition involving systemic muscular and joint pain

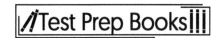

accompanied by fatigue. While researchers have yet to identify the cause, fibromyalgia is believed to be due to neurological problems with properly processing pain signals.

28. D: A client taking blood thinners may be hypertensive and/or at high risk for clotting. The therapist should ask more questions to determine whether massage is safe at the time.

29. D: Sodium bicarbonate, a very effective base, has the chief function to increase the pH of the chyme. Chyme leaving the stomach has a very low pH, due to the high amounts of acid that are used to digest and break down food. If this is not neutralized, the walls of the small intestine will be damaged and may form ulcers. Sodium bicarbonate is produced by the pancreas and released in response to pyloric stimulation so that it can neutralize the acid. It has little to no digestive effect.

30. A: All three joint types given are synovial joints, allowing for a fair amount of movement (compared with fibrous and cartilaginous joints). Of the three given, hinge joints, such as the elbow, permit the least motion because they are uniaxial and permit movement in only one plane. Saddle joints and condyloid joints both have reciprocating surfaces that mate with one another and allow a variety of motions in numerous planes, but saddle joints, such as the thumb carpal-metacarpal joint, allow more motion than condyloid joints. In saddle joints, two concave surfaces articulate, and in a condyloid joint, such as the wrist, a concave surface articulates with a convex surface, allowing motion in mainly two planes.

31. B: The power differential is a psychological term used to distinguish the dynamics in a relationship between two people based on roles such as teacher/student, employee/employer, and massage therapist/client. It is common for a client who feels positive results from massage therapy sessions to bestow a certain amount of power onto the massage therapist as someone who has the knowledge and skills to solve the client's problems. It is important for the massage therapist to acknowledge this power differentiation and never take advantage of the situation.

32. D: Both I & III are correct. It is true that proper table height allows the therapist to use appropriate body mechanics and avoid injury. Also, lower table heights allow for much greater pressure. There is no industry standard regulating what type of massage is appropriate for which table height; the main factor is the therapist's stature.

33. D: Hypertonic tissues possess excessive muscle tone due to tension and over-excitability of spindle fibers; hence, they are prone to painful spasms. Hypertonic tissues suffer from poor circulation and constricted range of motion, as the body allocates collagen to build scar tissue around the site of strain.

34. B: Yes, massage can help relieve stress. Although it cannot replace talk therapy, massage can go a long way in alleviating stress. Even for clients who are concerned about the time commitment of bodywork, massage lowers levels of cortisol, epinephrine, and norepinephrine in the body, while increasing levels of dopamine, serotonin, and oxytocin. This encourages a feeling of calm and well-being for the client regardless of their external stressors.

35. D: A dual relationship is any relationship with two distinct aspects. In massage therapy, one part of that is therapist/client; any other relationship between the same two people creates a dual relationship, whether it is therapist/family member, therapist/hairdresser, therapist/contractor, etc. Therapists are advised to be highly cautious in these situations, because an issue in one of the relationships could undoubtedly affect the other.

215

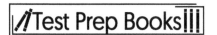

36. A: The three primary body planes are coronal, sagittal, and transverse. The coronal or frontal plane, named for the plane in which a corona or halo might appear in old paintings, divides the body vertically into front and back sections. The sagittal plane, named for the path an arrow might take when shot at the body, divides the body vertically into right and left sections. The transverse plane divides the body horizontally into upper or superior and lower or inferior sections. There is no medial plane, per se. The anatomical direction medial simply references a location close or closer to the center of the body than another location.

37. B: The smallest unit of a muscle fiber, a sarcomere, contains the actin and myosin proteins responsible for the mechanical process of muscle contractions. Located between two Z-lines, the actin and myosin filaments are configured in parallel, end-to-end, along the entire length of the myofibril. The sarcomere consists of four segments: the A-band, H-zone, I-band, and Z-line. The B-band and D-line are fictitious and are not components of a sarcomere.

38. A: Proprioception is the body's sense of limb position and orientation. Because Muscle Energy Technique uses both active and assisted (passive) stretching techniques, and passive range of motion often exceeds active ROM (especially post-isometric contraction), MET can help adjust a client's perception of their body.

Gentle circular friction of the large intestine in a clockwise direction facilitates digestion and is useful for clients with constipation and/or irritable bowel syndrome, while manual lymphatic drainage massage aids lymphatic circulation using gentle pressure to flush out waste.

All massage ideally induces a parasympathetic, or relaxed, state.

39. B: Acute pain is caused by injury; chronic pain lasts longer than 6 weeks. There are many differences between acute and chronic pain, but the main difference in their definitions is the timeline. Acute pain is caused by a specific injury, whereas chronic pain lasts longer than 6 weeks. Impact and injury can cause acute pain, while poor body mechanics (extremely common) can cause chronic pain. However, each type of pain can result from any number of injuries.

40. B: Very likely. In fact, the therapist should be extremely wary of any interviews that do away with the practical component. A practical interview is an essential part of any hiring process. The therapist should come prepared to perform a massage on their potential employer. This can be an awkward dynamic; the therapist's confidence under that pressure is a determining factor in whether they will get the job.

41. C: Yes, working on atrophied limbs can improve blood and lymph flow throughout the body. Atrophied limbs may not have strong or capable muscles, but the brain and heart continue to keep them alive with blood flow. Blood and lymph can pool in unused extremities, causing edema, pain, and poor circulation throughout the rest of the body. Massage is essential for relieving these symptoms.

42. D: Most bodily fluids, not including sweat. Standard precautions state that the therapist (or other healthcare provider) should avoid contact with most bodily fluids, such as blood, mucus, semen, vaginal secretions, saliva, etc. Sweat is not considered an infectious bodily fluid and will likely be encountered during massages.

43. C: Although the lungs may provide some cushioning for the heart when the body is violently struck, this is not a major function of the respiratory system. Its most notable function is that of gas exchange

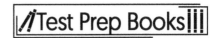

for oxygen and carbon dioxide, but it also plays a vital role in the regulation of blood pH. The aqueous form of carbon dioxide, carbonic acid, is a major pH buffer of the blood, and the respiratory system directly controls how much carbon dioxide stays and is released from the blood through respiration. The respiratory system also enables vocalization and forms the basis for the mode of speech and language used by most humans.

44. D: Muscle fibers, also called muscle cells (i.e., myocytes), are long, striated, cylindrical cells that are approximately the diameter of a human hair (50 to 100 μm); have many nuclei dispersed on the outside of the cell; and are covered by a fibrous membrane called the sarcolemma. Myofibrils, one of the smaller functional units within a myocyte, consist of long, thin (approximately 1 μm) chains of proteins. The smallest unit of a muscle fiber, a sarcomere, contains the actin and myosin proteins responsible for the mechanical process of muscle contractions.

45. D: Potassium, calcium, and sodium are electrolytes in the blood that carry electric charge and aid in muscle function. Sodium increases the volume of fluid in muscle cells; decreased sodium will cause the body to produce potassium, leading to decreased muscle volume. Nerve endings in muscle cells release calcium to signal the brain, causing muscular contraction and relaxation. Electrolyte imbalance can cause painful cramps and spasms. This is why regular hydration and a balanced diet are incredibly important to the health of muscle tissues.

46. B: Resting position is a brief moment of stillness at the beginning of a massage. This time allows the therapist and client to relax and begin communicating using touch instead of speech.

47. B: Transference is when a client develops feelings toward the therapist that are similar to feelings the client might have with someone outside of that professional relationship. Whether or not these are romantic feelings, they must be acknowledged and dealt with by the therapist. Countertransference is when the opposite happens and the therapist develops misplaced feelings towards the client.

48. C: An ancient holistic modality that involves placing needles at specific points in the body. Acupuncture is several thousand years old and was originally developed in China. Acupuncturists place needles at specific points in the body, prescribe herbs, and monitor their clients' progress. This is a holistic modality intended to treat body and mind together.

49. D: Overt sexual comments or advances from a client are unacceptable under any circumstances. The therapist should respond to this behavior by immediately terminating service and having the client removed from the premises. Massage therapists do meaningful and respected work that takes a good deal of education and training, and they should never be subjected to such demeaning behavior.

50. A: The forebrain contains the cerebrum, the thalamus, the hypothalamus, and the limbic system. The limbic system is chiefly responsible for the perception of emotions through the amygdala, while the cerebrum interprets sensory input and generates movement. Specifically, the occipital lobe receives visual input, and the primary motor cortex in the frontal lobe is the controller of voluntary movement. The hindbrain, specifically the medulla oblongata and brain stem, control and regulate blood pressure and heart rate.

217

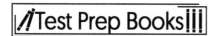
51. A: The sarcoplasmic reticulum is a network of tubular channels and vesicles that together provide structural integrity to the muscle fiber. The sarcoplasmic reticulum also acts as a calcium ion pump, moving Ca^{2+} ions from the sarcoplasm into the muscle fiber when the action potential reaches the cell. The Ca^{2+} binds with troponin, which causes the tropomyosin to move further into the double helix groove, allowing rapid binding of actin and myosin filaments and the power stroke that pulls the actin toward the center of the sarcomere, resulting in a contraction.

52. D: When working on a limb, the therapist should address the entire limb, starting and ending the session at the shoulder or the hip. This remains true even if the site of pain is at the distal end of the limb. Proximal/Distal/Proximal is a protocol which reminds the therapist to work on a limb in the following manner: First, the muscle tissue at the shoulder or hip joint is released, allowing blood to flow freely into the limb. Then, the therapist should work slowly down toward the site of injury, releasing all muscle tissue along the way. This is important because it leaves a clear path of blood vessels between the injury and the heart, which makes it possible for blood to flow easily to and from the area of pain. This limits the risk of edema and controls the natural inflammatory response.

53. B: Kyphosis, or rounding of the shoulders, often results from long hours spent hunched over a computer. It primarily compromises the SCM in the anterior neck, the erector spinae muscles running alongside the spine, the rhomboids, and the pectorals.

Swayback, more formally known as lordosis, refers to an anteriorly tilted pelvis that causes the gluteal muscles to protrude, contracting the lower back and weakening the hamstrings and abdominals. Knee hyperextension is often related to lordosis, while drop foot can be caused by tight hip abductors and dorsal extensors compromising the sciatic and peroneal nerves.

54. C: Although regulations for therapists vary from state to state, it is consistently true that therapists must receive an education from a legitimate and accredited school. The number of hours required depends on the location, but the program itself must be a qualifying one. It is best to check that a school is accredited before committing time and money to a massage therapy program.

55. B: Explain the history of aromatherapy and the client's different options. The client can only make an informed decision if they understand every detail of the recommended treatment. Informed consent is an important component of treatment, and the therapist should educate clients about new modalities. However, the therapist should bear the client's needs in mind. Some find it easier to follow an LMT's advice when they understand why it will help; others prefer to follow simple instructions without worrying about the details. It is best to offer clients enough options so they can make informed decisions, but not so many that they become overwhelmed. As a therapist, one cannot legally prescribe any course of treatment or medication.

56. B: Painkillers can damage the stomach, but there is no risk of addiction. This statement is false because many painkillers—particularly opiates—carry a high risk of addiction. The other statements are true. Painkillers indeed have short term benefits, but damage to the GI tract and addiction are among their long-term risks. NSAIDs, such as ibuprofen and aspirin, are available over the counter, while stronger medications require a prescription. Opiates carry the same Latin root as the illegal drug opium because they are derived from the same source. Legal versions of this drug are distilled further, so their effects are more specific and less powerful.

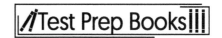

57. D: All of the above. Synergists are responsible for helping the primary movers or agonists carry out their specific movements. Synergists can help stabilize the point of origin of a muscle or provide extra pull near the insertion; in this sense, they can be considered "fixators." Some synergists can help prevent undesired movement at a joint. For example, for elbow flexion, the brachialis is a synergist to the biceps.

58. B: Choices I, II, and IV are correct. Here are examples of correct matches:

> Fibrous: sutures in skull
> Plane: intercarpal
> Saddle: thumb
> Hinge: elbow
> Condyloid: wrist
> Pivot: radial head on ulna
> Cartilaginous: pubic symphysis

59. C: Poor posture weakens certain muscle groups and forces others to compensate, often becoming hypertonic and resulting in decreased range of motion. Systemic muscle imbalance can result in an uneven gait.

60. D: All of the above. Overuse of heat therapy can result in overstimulation of the inflammatory response. Because inflammation is defined as the presence of heat, redness, swelling, and pain, this includes unnecessary pain. Although some pain is necessary in the healing process, because all healing includes inflammation, it is counterproductive to cause more pain than necessary. In severe cases, overuse of a heat pack or heating pad can indeed result in first-, second-, or third-degree burns.

61. B: Chair massage is a valuable way to promote massage therapy to the general public. The therapist can try setting up in an office or on a beach; the client does not need to disrobe, and passersby often want to learn more. Chair massage isn't the best strategy for prenatal work, as it puts too much pressure on the client's abdomen. It is rarely offered in medical settings, unless the clinic is running a promotion. The time of day has no bearing on the effectiveness of this modality.

62. A: Bruegger's Relief Position helps correct the forward head posture and medial rotation of the shoulders associated with kyphosis.

63. B: Energy work is a catch-all phrase used to describe any modality where the practitioner focuses on manipulating the client's alleged energy. Reiki is a popular form of this. Aromatherapy uses essential oils and scents to achieve physiological effects, but it is not a form of energy work.

64. D: Bony matrix is an intricate lattice of collagen fibers and mineral salts, particularly calcium and phosphorus. The mineral salts are strong but brittle, and the collagen fibers are weak but flexible, so the combination of the two makes bone resistant to shattering and able to withstand the normal forces applied to it.

65. C: Elbow extension and wrist flexion are movements that both take place in the sagittal plane. The sagittal plane cuts through the middle of the body dividing the body into right and left regions. Shoulder abduction and neck left tilt movements both occur in the frontal plane.

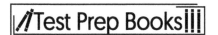

66. B: PROM is an acronym that therapists use to teach clients how to do certain rehab exercises. It is a more formal way of reminding them: "Try this exercise, but don't go too far. If it hurts, stop."

67. A: This is the number one rule when it comes to a massage therapist's scope of practice. Therapists do not diagnose. They can treat certain musculoskeletal conditions, but under no circumstances is a therapist to diagnose a client's problem. Protocol states that the therapist should merely suggest that the client see a physician to receive a proper diagnosis.

68. D: Insurance plans that have a low premium (the patient's monthly cost to carry the insurance) tend to have a higher deductible, unless most of the cost of the plan is covered by the patient's employer. High deductibles can be a barrier to patients seeking the treatment they need because they are responsible for all billed amounts until they've exceeded their deductible, after which point, the insurance coverage will start to kick in for services. Choice *A* refers to a copay. Choice *B* describes the insurance payment for a given procedure. Choice *C* describes the out-of-pocket maximum.

69. C: There is a high risk of miscarriage. Many believe it is a bad idea to even announce a pregnancy before the beginning of the second trimester since miscarriage during the first three months is so common. The question of whether massage is indicated during this time is a controversial one and depends on the advice of the supervising physician. However, to say it is "extremely dangerous" is a gross overstatement. Morning sickness, on the other hand, is most likely to occur toward the beginning of a pregnancy. The pubic symphysis does not separate during all pregnancies; if this does occur, it usually happens toward the end of the third trimester.

70. B: High levels of intoxication can affect blood pressure and result in arrhythmia. Because massage therapy increases circulation, it can also dangerously magnify the effects of alcohol and drugs. If a massage therapist suspects a client is under the influence, he or she should contact the supervisor.

71. A: The sternum is medial to the deltoid because it is much closer to (typically right on) the midline of the body, while the deltoid is lateral at the shoulder cap. Superficial means that a structure is closer to the body surface and posterior means that it falls behind something else. For example, skin is superficial to bone and the kidneys are posterior to the rectus abdominus.

72. B: Antagonists are muscles that oppose the action of the agonist—the primary muscle causing a motion. Hamstrings are the primary knee flexors—the agonists—and the quadriceps fire in opposition. The gastrocnemius does cross the knee joint, so it is a knee flexor, although secondary to the hamstrings. Tibialis anterior is on the shin and is involved in dorsiflexion.

73. B: Ask what exactly she is taking and research the effects of her prescriptions before performing massage. Herbs and supplements are powerful medicines. If a client is seeking treatment from an acupuncturist, the massage therapist should assume that the client has a very specific, long-term treatment plan designed to eliminate certain symptoms. It is essential for the therapist to learn what those symptoms are, how they are being treated, and how massage might interact with any other chemicals—even natural chemicals—in the client's system.

74. C: Yes, massage can directly improve a client's mental health. It is true that most effects of a massage are physical. However, any skin-to-skin contact—especially the prolonged touch of a trained professional—releases certain neurotransmitters in the brain. Massage increases serotonin, dopamine, and oxytocin levels. These chemicals are responsible for a person's sense of motivation, positive mental

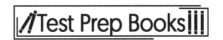

health, happiness, and their ability to bond with other people. Massage also decreases cortisol, the stress hormone. These chemical changes have a direct positive impact on mental and emotional health.

75. A: When the gluteus medius is not functioning properly, it can cause displacement of the hip during stance phase, when that side of the body is supporting weight. This is known as Trendelenburg's sign.

Arthritis is usually responsible for an arthrogenic gait, in which the hip is elevated to allow the toes to clear the ground. An ataxic or stumbling gait may indicate neurological problems or intoxication, which is a general contraindication to massage. Spasm in the psoas, responsible for hip flexion, can cause someone to appear bent at the waist and to demonstrate a psoatic limp.

76. C: Communication is essential in all relationships, but especially in massage therapy. Rules, regulations, and expectations must always be clearly articulated to therapists and any other employees. Entrepreneurs must be able to clearly communicate with clients and others in the business. Lack of communication is the cause of many misunderstandings and potentially harmful situations.

77. C: Politely suggest that he come back another day because massage is contraindicated when a client has a fever. Working on a client with a fever or flu-like symptoms is contraindicated for two reasons. First, the client exposes not only the therapist but all the therapist's other clients to the illness. Second, massage can dramatically exacerbate illness symptoms. By increasing circulation, massage can cause additional inflammation and spread infection throughout the body. Clients should heal from the illness on their own and seek massage once their symptoms subside.

78. C: Nociceptors are sensory receptors, mostly embedded in the dermis and epidermis, that specifically detect pain. They can sense pain in the forms of thermal, mechanical, or chemical stimulus, but these pain receptors are different from receptors that detect normal levels of stimulus. They carry the pain signals to the CNS via afferent sensory neurons. Temperature is detected via thermoreceptors, movement via mechanoreceptors and the entire proprioceptive and musculoskeletal systems, and vibration is detected by specialized mechanoreceptors, such as Ruffini endings.

79. A: The gentle movement of a client's joint by the therapist. During joint mobilizations, the therapist gently moves a client's joint through their pain-free range of motion. If a client experiences pain during this process, the therapist should immediately cease the technique. Note that the discomfort that comes with stretching tight muscles is normal.

80. A: Cortisol is a stress hormone released by the adrenal glands when the body is in the fight-or-flight response. Massage ideally induces a parasympathetic or relaxed state, in which the body can better attend to basic autonomic functions. The parasympathetic nervous system is responsible for digestion, breathing, and heart rate, all of which are compromised by stress.

81. C: Both A and B are correct. Skeletal muscles are muscles that a person can voluntarily move and are attached to bones. Smooth muscles, found in the digestive tract, behave very differently. Skeletal muscles are controlled by the somatic nervous system, whereas smooth muscles are controlled by the parasympathetic nervous system.

82. B: Tractioning techniques elongate the joints, most often along the spine, to help relieve back pain caused by muscle spasms, disc compression, or disc injury. Choice *A*, reflexology, is incorrect because this style of massage is applied to the feet. Choice *C*, reiki, is a form of energy work that is not specific to the back. Choice *D*, cryotherapy, involves the application of ice or ice packs to acute injuries to control

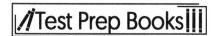

inflammation and decrease pain. While cryotherapy may be implemented with low back pain, it's not specific to back pain; in fact, cryotherapy has applications for many musculoskeletal injuries and pains, from foot issues to shoulder injuries.

83. C: HIPAA laws were designed to protect patient information as it moves electronically through third-party carriers such as insurance companies. Massage therapists are only held to HIPAA standards if their place of employment is considered a "covered entity," which is a place that deals with those third-party carriers. If the place of employment does not deal with insurance issues or medical records, then it would not fall under the HIPAA standards of practice.

84. A: No, it isn't. A client who recently took Advil (or any painkiller) should not receive massage. Painkillers make it impossible for the client to accurately sense what pressure is unbearably painful, which makes communication between the client and therapist difficult. More importantly, NSAIDs inhibit inflammation, so the massage will be ineffective while the effects of the drug last. As the NSAID wears off, any inflammation caused by the massage will kick in, and the client will experience unnecessary pain.

85. A: Fascia is fibrous connective tissue that envelops muscles and other organs. Like muscle fibers, fascia can become adhered and constricted at the site of injury or strain. Myofascial release and skin rolling help restore length and pliability to fascia. The other answers are invalid.

86. D: Protection, Rest, Ice, Compression, and Elevation. This acronym will alleviate much of the pain and inflammation caused by an acute injury. Pain-free movement through the range of motion prevents adhesions and scar tissue from forming. Rest gives the muscles a chance to heal slowly, without forcing other muscles to compensate. Ice controls the heat of inflammation, while compression and elevation both serve to alleviate swelling.

87. B: Even though spas and most private massage studios are not beholden to HIPAA standards, they should never be careless with clients' personal medical information. All intake forms and client notes should be kept in a locked file cabinet or on a password-protected computer. They should only be accessible to authorized individuals.

88. C: The therapist should breathe deeply. If the client hears this, it will inspire them to do the same. Humans have a natural tendency to match the breathing of people who are physically close to them. The therapist should breathe deeply for two reasons: to oxygenate their own muscles and care for their body and because deep and audible breathing invites the client to mimic their behavior. This encourages both people to relax and focus on the experience of physical touch. The client's body awareness will increase, and the therapist will have a clear sense of what work needs to be done.

89. D: Adrenergic drugs can be used during medical crises. Adrenergic drugs, such as an Epi-pen, are used to halt allergic reactions and asthma attacks. They contain one dose of epinephrine—another word for adrenaline. Cholinergic drugs are referred to as parasympathomimetics, not sympatholytics. Anticholinergic drugs relieve involuntary muscle spasms and do not stimulate muscle growth. Anticholinergic drugs block acetylcholine, decrease the fight-or-flight response, and are often used to treat GI disorders and asthma.

90. D: The principles of massage therapy include many of the positive benefits of massage such as increasing circulation, stretching and relieving tight muscles, and creating a healthy mind-body

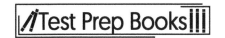

connection. The principles of massage are intended to improve the client's quality of life, both physically and mentally.

91. D: Positive rest position helps correct forward head posture and lordosis, both postural imbalances that cause the erector spinae muscles running alongside the spine to contract.

It is difficult to stretch the quadratus lumborum, but lying in a supine position with bent knees and placing a tennis ball beneath the QL can provide some relief. Bridges and low lunges with the posterior knee bent on the floor both stretch the hip flexors effectively. Reaching for one's toes, either while standing or sitting with the legs outstretched, is the classic antidote to tight hamstrings.

92. B: Invigorating. Tapotement, or percussive massage techniques, should stimulate the nerves in the area. This technique is not meant to bruise or injure the client, but it should "wake up" the surrounding muscle tissue. It is best applied to hypotonic or atrophied muscles, to stimulate growth and increase strength.

93. C: A latex barrier used to cover a single finger. Finger cots are used to protect the client and therapist when the therapist has a small wound, such as a papercut. They resemble latex gloves, though they only protect a single finger at a time.

94. A: This modality promotes the concept that the feet, particularly the plantar side of the feet, contain many pressure points that correspond to almost every part and operating system of the body. It is important to note that reflexology is not considered massage, but is often included on the menu of massage treatments at spas. It is common for a client to add a reflexology treatment to a massage service, but there are no massage techniques used during reflexology.

95. D: Wall angels alleviate medial rotation of the shoulders, stretching contracted pectoral muscles and strengthening the rhomboid muscles between the shoulder blades.

96. C: Massage therapy can be very beneficial if it is practiced correctly, but in the hands of an untrained person, it can be physically damaging. This is why education is so critical. There are contraindications to almost every modality, so a therapist must be well-informed about a client's unique health issues. Because massage therapy increases circulation, it can put extra pressure on blood vessels that might be constricted due to high blood pressure. Deep tissue massage can put further pressure on veins and vessels. Diabetes also causes circulatory problems, so the same vascular concerns are relevant. However, if these conditions are being treated by a physician, then these issues are much less of a concern to a therapist.

97. D: Effleurage, Petrissage, and Tapotement are the three main stroke techniques used in Swedish massage. Although other techniques such as friction and compression are also used, these are the defining techniques of Swedish massage.

98. A: A strain involves a damaged muscle or tendon; a sprain involves a damaged ligament. Strains and sprains can both be classified as Grade I, Grade II, or Grade III. Although many people use the words interchangeably, there is a very specific anatomical difference between the two types of injuries.

99. C: The gluteus medius plays an important role in stabilizing the pelvis while walking. When this muscle is weak, the IT bands—long sheaths of connective tissue on the outer thigh—may compensate, creating lateral force on the knee joint and pulling the patella outward.

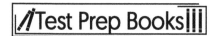

100. B: Hot stones should be heated in water to 120-150 degrees for a hot stone massage, although it is imperative that the therapist always cool and check the stones before applying them to the client's body. The therapist must communicate with the client throughout a hot stone massage to ensure comfort and safety.

Index

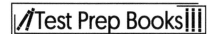

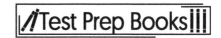

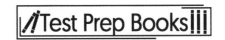

Sperm, 17, 24
Spermatocytes, 24
Spinal Cavity, 29
Spinal Column, 23, 49
Spinal Cord, 21, 22, 23, 27, 29, 38, 50, 61, 196, 211, 213
Spindle Fibers, 82, 215
Spleen, 11, 19, 29
Spongy Bone, 26, 27
Sports Massage, 74, 75, 82, 88, 110, 114, 199, 205, 214
Sprains, 52
Squamous, 18, 30
Stance Phase, 85, 86, 221
Standard Precautions, 49, 101, 102, 114, 201, 216
Steppage Gait, 86
Sternal Notch, 58
Sternum, 29, 39, 40, 42, 84, 85, 206
Stomach, 14, 15, 17, 29, 32, 33, 53, 63, 87, 195, 203, 212, 215, 218
Strains, 49, 51, 52, 223
Strains and Sprains, 52, 223
Stratified, 18, 30
Stretch Reflex, 38
Stroke, 35, 37, 50, 53, 72, 86, 209, 218, 223
Stroking, 72, 73
Subjective, 81, 84, 114, 196, 213, 214
Substantia Nigra, 22
Superficial, 19, 32, 48, 73, 82, 88, 111, 206, 220
Superior, 13, 32, 40, 42, 43, 214, 216
Superior Vena Cava, 13
Supine, 60, 77, 85, 87, 89, 103, 114, 196, 223
Suppressor T Lymphocytes, 18
Swayback, 85, 203, 210, 218
Sweat Glands, 19
Swing Phase, 85
Sympathetic Nerv, 23, 63, 64, 68, 87, 194, 211
Sympathetic Nervous System, 63, 64, 68, 87, 194, 211
Sympatholytic Drugs, 64, 208
Sympathomimetic Drugs, 64
Synergists, 20, 204, 219
Synovial Joints, 45, 215
Systemic Circulation, 13
Systole, 13
Systolic Blood Pressure (SBP), 13

T Tubules, 35
Tapotement, 72, 74, 100, 199, 209, 223
Temporal Lobe, 22
Temporomandibular Joint Dysfunction (TMJD), 53
Tendinitis, 52, 53, 83
Tendons, 19, 20, 30, 47, 76, 83, 113, 207, 214
Terminals, 20
Testes, 17, 24
Testes and Ovaries, 17
Testosterone, 17, 24
Thai Massage, 76
Thai Yoga Massage, 76
Thalamus, 22, 217
the Breath of Life, 79
Thermoreceptors, 27, 221
Third Degree Burns, 48
Thoracic, 29, 32, 39, 40, 42, 73
Thoracic Cavity, 29
Thymus Gland, 17
Thyroid Gland, 16, 58, 67
Tips, 103, 108, 109, 110, 114, 197, 214
Tissues, 11, 13, 16, 17, 19, 27, 29, 30, 47, 51, 77, 82, 102, 108, 214, 215
Topoisomerase Inhibitors, 65
Touch, 27, 35, 38, 48, 49, 51, 58, 60, 61, 69, 70, 71, 72, 79, 84, 87, 90, 92, 93, 107, 109, 110, 111, 112, 113, 202, 203, 206, 212, 217, 220, 222
Trabeculae, 27
Trachea, 25, 29
Traction, 72, 73, 101, 112, 114
Transference, 93, 202, 217
Transitional, 30, 45
Transverse, 16, 30, 35, 39, 40, 42, 84, 200, 208, 216
Transverse Plane, 31, 84, 216
Transverse-Tubular System, 35
Treatment Plan, 49, 109, 112, 113, 114, 115, 214, 220
Trendelenburg Gait, 86
Tricuspid Valve, 13, 214
Tricyclic Antidepressants, 63
Trigger Point Therapy, 51, 53, 58, 68, 73, 87, 88
Trigger Point Therapy (TRPT), 58
Trigger Points, 58, 73, 74, 87, 209
Tropomyosin, 35, 36, 218

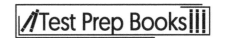

Dear MBLEx Test Taker,

We would like to start by thanking you for purchasing this study guide for your MBLEx exam. We hope that we exceeded your expectations.

Our goal in creating this study guide was to cover all of the topics that you will see on the test. We also strove to make our practice questions as similar as possible to what you will encounter on test day. With that being said, if you found something that you feel was not up to your standards, please send us an email and let us know.

We would also like to let you know about other books in our catalog that may interest you.

NASM

This can be found on Amazon: amazon.com/dp/1637757735

ACSM CPT

amazon.com/dp/1637754477

We have study guides in a wide variety of fields. If the one you are looking for isn't listed above, then try searching for it on Amazon or send us an email.

Thanks Again and Happy Testing!
Product Development Team
info@studyguideteam.com

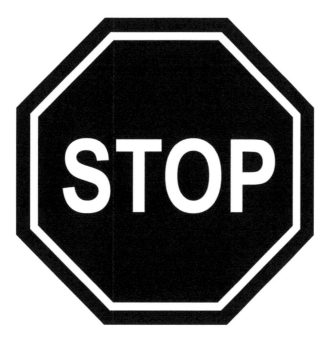

FREE Test Taking Tips Video/DVD Offer

To better serve you, we created videos covering test taking tips that we want to give you for FREE. **These videos cover world-class tips that will help you succeed on your test.**

We just ask that you send us feedback about this product. Please let us know what you thought about it—whether good, bad, or indifferent.

To get your **FREE videos**, you can use the QR code below or email freevideos@studyguideteam.com with "Free Videos" in the subject line and the following information in the body of the email:

   a. The title of your product

   b. Your product rating on a scale of 1-5, with 5 being the highest

   c. Your feedback about the product

If you have any questions or concerns, please don't hesitate to contact us at info@studyguideteam.com.

Thank you!